Delivering Neonatal Care

The Neonatal Unit as a Working Environment: A Survey of Neonatal Unit Nursing

M. E. Redshaw

A. Harris

J. C. Ingram

Institute of Child Health
University of Bristol

618.9201 RED

ISBN 0 11321940 7

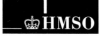

Published by HMSO and available from:

HMSO Publications Centre
(Mail, fax and telephone orders only)
PO Box 276, London SW8 5DT
Telephone orders 0171 873 9090
General enquiries 0171 873 0011
(queuing system in operation for both numbers)
Fax orders 0171 873 8200

HMSO Bookshops
49 High Holborn, London WC1V 6HB
(counter service only)
0171 873 0011 Fax 0171 831 1326
68–69 Bull Street, Birmingham B4 6AD
0121 236 9696 Fax 0121 236 9699
33 Wine Street, Bristol BS1 2BQ
0117 9264306 Fax 0117 9294515
9–21 Princess Street, Manchester M60 8AS
0161 834 7201 Fax 0161 833 0634
16 Arthur Street, Belfast BT1 4GD
01232 238451 Fax 01232 235401
71 Lothian Road, Edinburgh EH3 9AZ
0131 228 4181 Fax 0131 229 2734
The HMSO Oriel Bookshop
The Friary, Cardiff CF1 4AA
01222 395548 Fax 01222 384347

HMSO's Accredited Agents
(see Yellow Pages)

and through good booksellers

Contents

Preface

The Department of Health is to be congratulated for their wisdom in commissioning this study of care in Neonatal Units. Neonatology is a specialist area of practice which has evolved at an amazing rate in recent years. What applied twenty years ago, no longer obtains. Up to date information on the service was much needed and will provide a point of comparison for the future.

The capabilities of teams in these specialised centres have mushroomed and advancing technology has made the impossible possible. Even smaller and sicker babies are now kept alive. But this success story has its dark side and lurking in the backgroud are perplexing questions. Is the possible desirable? Is the staffing level adequate to deal with the increasingly sophisticated machinery, the psycho-social needs of relatives and the intensive nature of the hands-on care of the babies? Can society cope with the end result of such life saving? These and many other anxieties add to the burden carried by staff in this specialised area of care.

Changes in the organisation of the Health Service and of the medical and nursing professions have put pressure on individuals to take on more and more responsibility for their own professional development as well as maintaining standards in their clinical practice. It requires dedication and energy beyond the normal confines of the working day to stay abreast of progress and to offer the kind of humanitarian care which society as well as colleagues have come to expect of these professionals. When neither managers nor the purse-holders appear to recognise the pressures and emotional drain, it is all too easy for staff in Neonatal Units to feel undervalued and misunderstood. Many areas of caring have their share of stress but, in neonatal intensive care, superimposed on the common elements is the added burden occasioned by dealing with families who are coping with profound anxiety and grief at a time when happiness and congratulations are the norm.

This report uncovers something of the complexity of working with sick neonates and their families. It will reassure staff in these units to see that their stresses are recognised and understood. It will allow others to appreciate not only something of the source of these stresses and the levels of anxiety and depression experienced, but also something of the satisfaction which the staff and the parents report. The aim of the study was, indeed, a positive one: to enhance the quality of the care in paediatric and neonatal intensive care units. With its clear explanation of the study design and methods, a detailed account of the findings and useful summaries of the main points, this report provides the essential base to realise that purpose. I commend it to clinicians, managers and educators alike.

Hazel E McHaffie
October 1995

Foreword

The Strategy for Research in Nursing asserts that there is little merit in fostering research if it is to reach only a small audience (DOH, 1993). The need for research-based practice has been recognised and is supported by the Department of Health. The dissemination process is seen as a vital and healthy part of a vigorous research process which must include practitioners, clinicians, managers and academics. The present study was commissioned and funded by the Department of Health which also supported the dissemination process by providing funding for an additional year during which an executive summary was prepared and presentations made to a range of professional groups. A follow-up to this has been the preparation by the research team of an expanded version of the full study report, containing additional and updated material to be circulated on a wider scale.

Acknowledgements

We owe a great debt to all the nurses, doctors and parents who participated in the study and would like to express our thanks to them. We would also like to thank the senior nursing and medical staff who facilitated data collection and our hospital visits. Mike Taysum, Karen Birmingham, Nandi Simpson and Tina Owen contributed computing, data entry and coding skills. Assistance with the multivariate analyses came from Peter Cripps and Kenton Morgan. We are also grateful to Miranda Mugford, Glyn Russell and Lin McDonagh who commented on the full report.

Advice and support have generously been given throughout the project by the following members of the Project Advisory Group:

Professor J. D. Baum, Director, Institute of Child Health.

Dr P. J. Fleming, Consultant Neonatologist, Bristol.

Dr N. Marlow, Consultant Paediatrician, Bristol.

Dr K. Thorpe, Psychologist, Institute of Child Health.

Miss M. Colbeck, Senior Nurse, Neonatal Unit, St Michaels Hospital, Bristol.

Professor P. Dunn, British Association of Perinatal Medicine.

Professor J. Golding, Epidemiology, Institute of Child Health

Dr M. Woolridge, Research Fellow, Institute of Child Health.

Mrs P. Hale, Representative of Neonatal Nurses Association.

Dr T. Marteau, Psychologist, Royal Free Hospital, London.

Dr E. Scott, Liaison Officer, Department of Health.

Miss J. Greenwood, Department of Health.

The Department of Health commissioned, funded and supported the project for the full duration of the study and many thanks are due to Dr Elizabeth Scott in her role as liaison officer.

Chapter 1 · Introduction

The Specialty of Neonatal Care

The setting of standards in health care, the development of guidelines and indicators for quality, changes in nursing roles and working practices are all elements in neonatal nursing today and in nursing more generally (DOH, 1992a, 1992b, 1993, 1994; CSAG, 1993; Audit Commission, 1993; 1995). The rationale for a study of neonatal nursing came from two different perspectives. The first originated in concerns about fundamental issues intrinsic to the work of neonatal care and the links with occupational stress occurring in this kind of environment. The work situation of neonatal care, intensive in nature and with exposure to death and abnormality and families in extreme distress, contrasts with the more usual environment associated with normal births and caring for healthy newborn infants with their mothers. It also has elements that are common to other work situations and other caring professions. The other perspective centred on current issues arising from the present organization and structure of the neonatal service. The key concerns and problems in this area are currently those associated with staffing levels, changes in skill mix, training needs and effectiveness. The experiences and perceptions of nursing staff and parents as individuals in the testing environment of neonatal care are also an essential focus of concern from the consumer viewpoint, that of the professional carers and of the purchasing authorities. Thus, a need was recognised for an accurate, data-based picture of the present situation in the specialty and an assessment of the direction and potential for change. This was considered particularly important at a time of rapid evolution in the health service, when many possibilities for new developments in organisational structure and models of care are being considered.

Background

Increasing interest and research in the area of perinatal medicine and neonatal care has largely centred on changes in clinical practice. Research questions have ranged widely, but have focused on subjects such as breech delivery for preterm infants, the use of ultrasound, methods of caring for extremely low birth weight babies and the benefits of surfactant. The needs of the small patients and their families experiencing the delivery of care have also been considered, with greater awareness of the effects of hospital environments on parents and babies (Davis et al, 1983; Redshaw, Rivers and Rosenblatt, 1985).

Less attention has been directed towards organisational aspects of this segment of the health care system and the needs and work experiences of the staff working in it.

More recently within the health service the need for research on the areas of organisation, management, job content and satisfaction has been recognised. There have been research reports on the implications of medical staffing structures in obstetrics (Green, Kitzinger, and Coupland, 1986) and paediatric intensive care (British Paediatric Association, 1993) the interface between nurses and junior medical staff (Greenhalge, 1994), the roles of nurses and technicians in high technology clinical areas (Youngman, Mockett and Baxter, 1988), and the numbers, qualifications and training of nurses working in high technology care (Department of Health Report, 1989). A Report of the Royal College of Physicians on the organisation of medical care for the newborn (RCP, 1988) discussed many of the concerns in the overlapping areas of neonatal paediatrics and obstetrics. More recently, the House of Commons Maternity Services Committee Report (1992) and report on "Changing Childbirth" (1993) have covered similar ground with a different emphasis. Increasingly too, attention is being paid to the problem of occupational stress in health service workers (Rees and Cooper, 1992) including hospital nurses (Tyler and Cushway, 1992). However, quantitative research and data collection, specifically on the structure and the organisation of many areas of care, seen from the nursing and medical points of view has largely been absent.

The kind of nursing and medical work carried out in neonatal units has changed dramatically over recent decades. A high degree of technical skill is required, in conjunction with skill and sensitivity in interpersonal behaviour and caretaking (Bellig, 1980; Boxall and Garcia, 1983; Jacobson, 1983). Stress is a common feature of many job situations, but those working in hospital environments seem particularly vulnerable, owing to the nature of the work undertaken (Parkes, 1985; Hingley and Cooper, 1986; Payne and Firth-Cozens, 1987). The rapid advances in technology, which are part of modern medical care have affected the way neonatal medicine is practised and the development of neonatal intensive care nursing. In association with this, there has been some interest expressed in the way that medical and nursing personnel function in complex settings where there is a constant threat of crisis that demands discriminating perception and skill in relating to infants, parents and machines (Bender, 1981; Sherman, 1980; Walker, 1982; Jacobson, 1983). Despite this interest, relatively few large scale empirical studies have been carried out on the work experiences and characteristics of staff working in these demanding environments (Payne and Firth-Cozens, 1987).

"Stress" and "burnout" are commonly accepted terms used in describing the longterm effects of working in the environment of neonatal care (Marshall and Kasman, 1980), but there has been little quantitative data collection and analysis of the factors involved (Frader, 1979; Astbury and Yu, 1980). Against a background of the constant strain of coping with their own and other feelings of distress, there are unexpected deaths that may affect staff acutely (Clarke et al, 1984). Other major sources of stress are found in conflicts involving

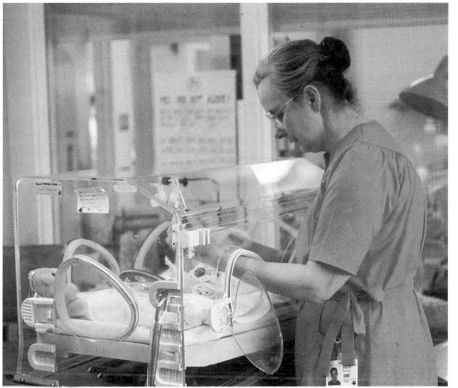

An experienced neonatal nurse caring for a sick and ventilated baby

philosophical and ethical issues (Gustaitis and Young, 1986; Guillemin and Holmstrom, 1986) and in the professional relationships within and between teams of nursing and medical staff (Hingley and Cooper, 1986).

The Aims of the Study

The delivery of front-line care in an acute sector of the health care system, the neonatal service, was the focus of this investigation. A three year research project was commissioned and funded by the Department of Health and carried out independently by the Institute of Child Health in the University of Bristol. The aim was to initiate a major study that could inform policy and identify possible improvements in practice and organisation in the context of concerns about stress in neonatal nursing, issues of staffing, skill mix and training. The study could also provide a point of comparison with other areas of nursing and medicine and perhaps more importantly, could be used as a reference point over time, following innovation and modification to the patterns of care provision.

The objective was to carry out a large-scale study of neonatal nursing in England; to document and examine some of the specific issues raised in relation to the organisation and management of neonatal units. Common features of neonatal care as it is practised and differences and similarities between units were to be used to illustrate the degree to which there is consensus, conformity and innovation in this area. The organisational features to be investigated included nursing and medical staffing, the skill mix in operation, staff education and training and management style and structure.

The responsibility which nursing staff carry for the care of small, sick babies may be both a rewarding and a costly one in personal as well as other terms. To this end a thorough investigation was planned of the psychological and organisational factors that may enable the needs of the nurses working in this situation to be more effectively met. The aim was to describe the psycho-social and other characteristics of nursing staff working in a large number of differently sized units and aspects of the work situation, and to link these with data on levels of anxiety, depression and perceived sources of stress and satisfaction. Parental perceptions and experiences in the same neonatal units were also to be investigated.

In the longer term, a wider goal lay in raising awareness of the pertinent issues and in providing information that could be used by individual units and hospitals in assessing their own situation and performance. Implicit in this goal was the aim of assisting in the raising of standards, enhancing the quality of care, and in improving selection, training and support for nursing staff in these and other types of paediatric and intensive care units.

References

Astbury, J. and Yu, V. H. Y. (1982). Determinants of stress for staff in a neonatal intensive care unit. Arch. Dis. Childhood, 57, 108.

Audit Commission (1993) Children First. HMSO London.

Audit Commission (1995) The Doctors' Tale: Report on Medical Staffing. HMSO. London.

Bellig, L. (1980). The expanded nursing role in the neonatal intensive care unit. *Clinics in Perinatology*, 7, 159–171.

Bender, H. (1981). Experiences in running a nursing staff group in a hospital intensive care unit. *J. Child Psychotherapy*, 7, 20–28.

Boxall, J. and Garcia, J. (1983). Stress and the nurse in neonatal units. *Midwives Chronicle*, 407–410.

British Paediatric Association (1993) The Care of Critically Ill Children. Report of the Working Party on Paediatric Intensive Care. BPA. London.

Clarke, T. A., Maniscalco, W. M., Taylor-Brown, S., Roghman, K. J., Shapiro, D. L. and Hannon-Jackson, G. (1984). Job satisfaction and stress among neonatologists. *Paediatrics* 74, 52–57.

Clinical Standards Advisory Group (1993) Access and Availability of Specialist Services. HMSO London.

Davis, J. A., Richards, M. P. M. and Roberton, N. R. C.(1983) Parent-baby Attachment in Premature Infants. London, Croom Helm.

Department of Health (1989). Survey of Nurses in High Technology Care. NHSME.

Department of Health (1992) Patient's Charter, HMSO, London.

Department of Health (1992) Health of the Nation, HMSO, London.

Department of Health (1993) A Vision for the Future: The Nursing, Midwifery, and Health Visiting Contribution to Health and Health care. NHSME. HMSO, London.

Department of Health (1994) The Challenges of Nursing and Midwifery in the 21st Century. DOH, London.

Department of Health Expert Maternity Group (1993) Changing Childbirth. HMSO, London.

Frader J. E. (1979). Difficulties in providing intensive care. *Paediatrics*, **64**, 10–16.

Green, J., Kitzinger, J. and Coupland, V. (1986) The Division of Labour: Implications of medical staffing structures for midwives and doctors on the labour ward. Report of Child Care and Development Group, Cambridge.

Greenhalge and Company (1994) The Interface Between Junior Doctors and Nurses. Report for the Department of Health. Greenhalge, Macclesfield.

Guillemin, J. H. and Holmstrom, L. L. (1986) Mixed Blessings: Intensive Care for Newborns. Oxford University Press, Oxford.

Gustaitis, R. and Young, E. W. D. (1986). A Time to be Born and a Time to Die: Conflicts and Ethics in an Intensive Care Unit. Addison Wesley, Reading, Massachusetts.

Hingley, P. and Cooper, C.(1986) Stress and the Nurse Manager. Wiley, Chichester.

House of Commons Health Committee Report. Maternity Services, (1992), Volume I, HMSO, London.

Jacobson, S. F. (1983). Stresses and coping strategies of neonatal intensive care nurses. *Research in Nursing and Health*, **6**, 33–40.

Marshall, R. E. and Kasman, C. (1980) Burn-out in the neonatal intensive care unit. *Paediatrics*, **65**, 1161–1165.

Parkes, K. R. (1985). Stressful episodes reported by first-year student nurses. *Social Science Medicine*, **20**, 945–953.

Payne, R. and Firth-Cozens, J. (1987) Stress in Health Professionals. Wiley, Chichester.

Redshaw, M. E., Rivers, R. P. A. and Rosenblatt, D. B. (1985). Born Too Early. Special Care for Your Preterm Baby. Oxford University Press, Oxford.

Rees, D. and Cooper, C. L. (1992) Occupational stress in health service workers in the UK. *Stress Medicine*, **8**, 79–90.

The Royal College of Physicians. (1988) Medical Care of The Newborn in England and Wales. RCP, London.

Sherman, M. (1980). Psychiatry in the neonatal intensive care unit. *Clinics in Perinatology*, 7, 33–46.

Tyler, P. and Cushway, D. (1992) Stress, coping and mental wellbeing in hospital nurses. *Stress Medicine*, **8**, 91–98.

Walker, C. (1982) Neonatal intensive care and stress. *Archives of Disease in Childhood*, **57**, 85–88.

Youngman, M., Mockett, S. and Baxter, C.(1988). The Roles of Nurses and Technicians in High Technology Areas, Preliminary Report, DHSS, London.

Chapter 2 · Study Design and Methodology

Introduction

The study set out to be an essentially descriptive one, aiming to document many aspects of the working environment of neonatal units, focusing on a wide range of organisational and individual experiential factors.

The hospital setting presents a challenge to the observer or researcher: hospitals have a distinct culture, with their own perspectives, goals, rules, and language that are very different from other areas of life. This is as true of the neonatal unit as other specialised areas of care. The first objective was to collect general information in the form of basic "unit profiles" from a large number of neonatal units. These were to provide a substantial contextual background for the second and third phases, in which the focus was on the experiences and perceptions of individual nurses and parents.

The Study Design

A three stage process for data collection was adopted. The over all design and organisation of the project is illustrated in Figure 2.1.

During Phase I four neonatal units in each of the 14 health regions of England (those in operation until April 1994) were selected (a regional centre, a sub-regional centre and two district units), resulting in a total of 56 that were asked to participate. The definitions of these types of unit are as described in the Report of the Royal College of Physicians (1988). The units were chosen by the research team without reference to the advisory group and in advance of the study. They were selected to provide a widely distributed, yet balanced, nationally representative sample in terms of size, geographical location and the population served. The numbers of cots in an individual unit ranged from 7–30, and in a combined service the highest number was 45. In choosing a regional and sub-regional unit from each of the fourteen health regions, the whole sample is slightly more biased towards larger units, when compared with the Department of Health survey of nurses working in high technology care (1989). In the present study, with its focus on neonatal nursing as a developing specialty, it would not have been appropriate to have included the smallest peripheral units. Such units typically have very few cots, are often closed and when open are staffed by midwives from the maternity unit. All the units originally selected participated in Phase I of the study. Two units subsequently

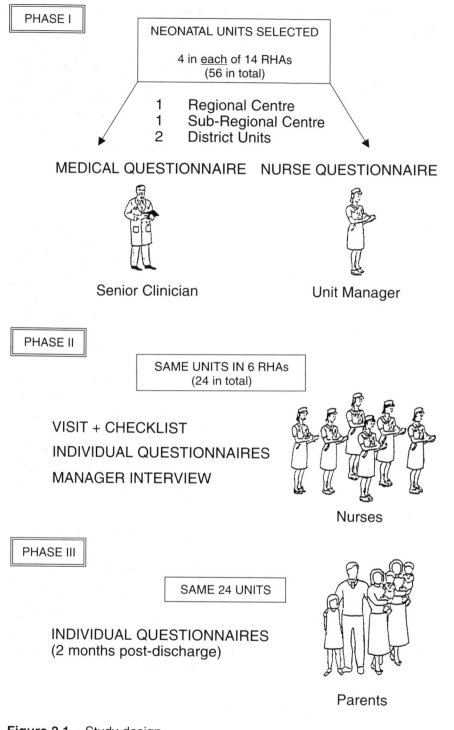

PHASE I

NEONATAL UNITS SELECTED

4 in each of 14 RHAs
(56 in total)

1   Regional Centre
1   Sub-Regional Centre
2   District Units

MEDICAL QUESTIONNAIRE   NURSE QUESTIONNAIRE

Senior Clinician   Unit Manager

PHASE II

SAME UNITS IN 6 RHAs
(24 in total)

VISIT + CHECKLIST

INDIVIDUAL QUESTIONNAIRES

MANAGER INTERVIEW

Nurses

PHASE III

SAME 24 UNITS

INDIVIDUAL QUESTIONNAIRES
(2 months post-discharge)

Parents

Figure 2.1 · Study design

changed size and status and comparable alternatives were selected from the same region.

Amongst the selected units at regional level, were three that could be described as "mega" units. Two of these were running two slightly differently sized neonatal units together as one service. The data used from these units relate to the combined service, though if a specific facility under consideration was different, the data from the larger, more intensive unit were used. The third "mega" unit occurred where medical and surgical facilities for newborns were organised separately, with separate nursing establishments, and here the medical unit data were used.

Unit Data Collection

In setting up the study, introductory letters were initially sent to regional nurses and those responsible for maternity services in the district health authorities and hospitals concerned. Senior medical and nursing staff responsible for neonatal care in the selected units were sent letters and project information sheets in July 1990, three months prior to requests for information. Subsequently each unit approached was sent two questionnaires: one directed to the senior nursing manager responsible for the unit and the other to the senior clinician responsible for the medical management. The confidentiality of the replies was emphasised.

The data requested in the nursing questionnaire included the location and type of unit, staffing establishment and vacancies, grades of staff employed, those qualified in the specialty, vacancies and sickness figures. The medical questionnaire was designed in two parts, the first of which included details of medical staffing, medical cover, responsibilities in other departments and location of the unit in relation to the other departments. Much of the information requested in the second part of the medical questionnaire concerned the population of babies admitted and the medical statistics for the previous year. As in some cases these were not available at the time, the option was given of returning the unit statistics separately when they had been collated and became available.

Questionnaires were sent out with stamped addressed return envelopes and reminders six weeks later. Continued non-response was followed by a telephone call. Most of the returned questionnaires were filled in and returned within an eight week period. Since some questions required checking through records, it was not possible to specify a time period by which the information was required. However, answers to questions about statistics or unit policy were unlikely to be affected by minor variations in timing of response.

Obtaining Ethical Permission

The Department of Health guidelines (DOH, 1991; Neuberger, 1992) emphasise the importance of medical research, the responsibility of the National Health Service in supporting research and the role of a local research ethics committee in advising on the ethics of research using human subjects. As a multi-centre study the same research proposal was submitted to 24 district health authority ethical committees in the different areas where the units were located. The objective was to obtain permission for the second and third stages of study which required the participation of individual nurse and parent subjects.

The process was informative, if time-consuming. Many aspects of ethical committee processing varied, including the forms, information required, timing and decision-making, reflecting individual factors and local situations. Sixteen of the 24 DHAs had a specific form for submission; five required that it be supplemented by a full protocol and the remainder required a protocol without a form. Additional information was requested by ten committees and four invited attendance at the relevant meeting. The length of the form ranged from 1–10 pages, between one and nineteen copies of the application form were required by the different committees and up to twelve copies of the parents' letters and questionnaires. Letters of local support were requested by nine of the 24 committees, most commonly from hospital consultants in the target hospitals.

The time required for processing varied such that the lag between submission and approval ranged from 22–298 days, with a mean of 109 days. Delays were in some instances the result of consulting parent advisors, though for six of the submissions these were associated with local management or personnel problems, rather than with specific ethical problems in the proposed research. Fourteen committees gave approval without modification and three rejected the proposal initially. Six requested minor modifications to the wording of parents' letters, different in each case. Alterations to the subject groups were requested by three committees based in district general hospitals: two wished the parents whose babies had died to be left out and one requested that no parents take part at all. In the first two cases there were no deaths within the period for which data were collected and so there was no effect of this request on the study. In the third case the research team agreed that no parents be contacted at all, though data were collected on individual nurses. Another committee insisted on a procedural change in the method of contacting parents, involving local hospital medical and nursing staff. Apprehension about parental involvement in the research was the most frequently voiced concern, even from committees giving permission. The positive response of parents themselves would tend to suggest that the anxiety expressed may have been overstated, at least in relation to this fairly straightforward consumer part of the survey. (See sections on Parent Data Collection & Returns).

Nurse Data Collection

A sub-sample of 24 units from the 56 participating in the first phase of the study was selected and took part in the second stage. As with Phase I, a balance was maintained in terms of geographical location and the population served. The same four units from each of six widely distributed English Health Regions as had participated in the first stage of the data collection were contacted. All the nursing staff involved in 'hands on' care for babies or directly responsible for neonatal unit management were included in the study.

In order to reach individual nurses working in these units each unit was contacted and then visited by two members of the research team. The timing of visits was to a great extent dependent on obtaining ethical committee permission for the study to go ahead. In the course of each visit the team were shown round the unit, introduced to the staff working there and were available to meet and talk to those working on the different shifts. The duration of visits ranged from 9–14 hours and, where necessary, the team could return the following day. Staff lists had been obtained in advance and individually addressed letters and questionnaire packs were prepared and left for each member of the nursing staff to complete and return directly in their own time in a prepaid envelope. If necessary, after four weeks, a different letter and another copy of the questionnaire were sent individually, after which no further requests for participation were made. Neither unit nor hospital management were involved in encouraging or ensuring data return.

A mixture of structured and open-ended questions were used in the individual nurse questionnaire which also contained a number of standard instruments used in other studies (Hingley and Cooper, 1986; Spelton et al, 1993) (see Table 2.1.). A wide range of topics were covered that included a nurse's work experience, education, training, details of their current post and work, health and wellbeing, perceptions of the working environment and concerns about working in this specialty. A pilot study, using a first version of the questionnaire with 111 nurses, 89 of whom responded (82%), indicated that the general design was satisfactory and that few modifications were required.

Throughout the study, confidentiality was of the utmost importance. Rigorous professional guidelines were followed: numbered questionnaires were used; data were made anonymous and entered on the project computer system and data in any form were only accessible to the research team. At each hospital visit, during which nurses on the different shifts were seen, these points were stressed to the manager and others being asked to participate.

Parent Data Collection

Parents, whose babies had been cared for in 23 of the same 24 units from which nursing staff had been recruited, were the focus for the third part of the study. A completely unselected group were recruited by including all families whose babies had stayed at least 48 hours on the target units and had been discharged in the six week period immediately prior to the project team's visit. A small number of subjects were lost (7) where babies had been transferred to another unit or paediatric ward and were then only discharged following a further long stay (3 months or more). In these cases the perceptions of what might have been a relatively short stay in the target unit could have been coloured by the subsequent exposure to hospital care in another context. Two further babies who were no longer being cared for by their own parents were not included, nor

Table 2.1 · List of data collected on individual nurses

Nature of the work	Task inventory:
	Responsibilities
	Tasks:
	    basic infant care
	    helping parents
	    general duties
	    management and organisation
	    teaching and training
	
	Types of babies cared for
	Technical tasks
	Assistance with medical procedures
	"Extended" role tasks

Individual circumstances	Current work situation Educational background and Training Personal circumstances Social support Life events list Type A behaviour (Bortner and Rosenman,1967)
Stress	Nurse Stress Index (Harris, Hingley and Cooper,1988) Sources of stress Stressful incidents
Health	General health and fitness Illness checklist Sickness information
Psychological wellbeing	General Health Questionnaire (Goldberg and Williams, 1988)
Attitudes to neonatal care	Perceptions of the neonatal unit Issues and concerns in neonatal care

was one family whose baby had died and about whom the senior medical staff felt considerable concern. A total of 539 families were recruited.

Admission and discharge books and other unit documentation, as well as computerised record systems were used to identify the subjects and collect a small amount of basic information. This included date of birth, sex of baby, type of delivery, gestation, birthweight, reasons for admission and contact address of the mother. Details of any transfers were also taken. Only the very small number of subjects meeting the criteria that were referred to above were excluded from the study at this stage.

Parents were sent a letter and a questionnaire two months after their baby had been discharged home. A pilot study with 40 mothers, 30 of whom responded (75%) indicated that only minor adjustments were required to the questionnaire. This part of the study was concerned with parents' experiences and perceptions of the neonatal service and so no standard psychological instruments were used. The topics covered by the questionnaire included basic demographic information, details of the pregnancy, birth, involvement in care, the facilities used, attitudes towards the neonatal unit (NNU) and about going home. A mixture of structured and open-ended questions, including adjective checklists, was used.

Data Returns

Details of the subject numbers for the different parts of the study and the associated returns are shown in Table 2.2.

The nursing questionnaire used in Phase I was returned by all 56 units. A total of 82% of senior clinicians returned Part 1 of the medical questionnaire (46 out of 56) and 64% (36 out of 56) Part 2. A number of units appeared slow to compile statistics, some were unable to collect them in a manageable format and others may have been reluctant to pass them on. Some statistical information was obtained at district level from perinatal reports and the Office of Population Censuses and Surveys. Additional information was also obtained in the course of visits. However in many instances, the variable quality of data collection on site, delays in compiling adequate statistics for annual reports and a reluctance to facilitate comparisons have contributed to a less than complete data set for this part of the study.

During Phase II, 929 nurses were recruited in the main study group 724 of whom replied (78%) and 718 of whom completed and returned the questionnaire. Of the 929, eight were male nurses (0.9%) and four of these returned questionnaires. The sample of individual nurses from the twenty-four units was found, with very minor differences, to be representative of the 1890 employed

Table 2.2 · Subject numbers and response rates for the three different stages in the study

Stages	Subjects	Timing	Response Rates
Phase I	56 units (1890 nurses)	Autumn 1990	Clinicians Part I 82% Part II 64% Nurse Managers 100%
Phase II	24 units (929 nurses)	June 1991–April 1992 Questionnaire left at visit	Individual Nurses 78% (718 completed)
Phase III	23 units (539 parents 575 babies)	Questionnaire posted 2 months post-discharge Born May 1991–April 1992	Individual parents 80% (432 parents 456 babies) (Including bereaved parents)

in the fifty-six units as a whole. As Table 2.3a. and 2.3b. show, a comparison of the proportions at the different grades and from the different types of unit shows them to be very similar.

A breakdown of the responders and non-responders by grade and title is given in Table 2.4a and 2.4b. The distribution of these by title and grade was largely similar, with the staff at lower grades being slightly less likely to respond, though not significantly so.

In Phase III parents of the surviving babies had been recruited from 23 of the same 24 units and a high response rate of 80% was achieved with this subject group. A total of 444 completed questionnaires were returned from families with surviving babies. As only 24 out of the 36 parents with twins responded (67%), this group may have been slightly under-represented. In the other respects examined the babies and families of those who did not respond appeared to differ little from those who participated: the gestational age at birth was not significantly different, neither was the type of delivery nor reasons for admission. Hospital data on maternal age was often absent and though there may have been a difference, it was not possible to compare the two groups in this respect.

Table 2.3a · Sample Characteristics by Grade

Grade	All Nurses Phase I (Source: Unit Management 56 units, n=1890) %	Nurses Phase II (Source: Nurses 24 units, n=718) %
A	5.56	2.09
B	5.24	5.71
C	8.73	8.77
D	11.75	9.19
E	30.79	32.45
F	15.71	18.80
G	18.94	17.97
H	1.8	3.48
I	1.48	1.53

Table 2.3b · Sample Characteristics by Unit Type

	All Nurses Phase I (Source: Unit Management 56 units, n=1890) %	Nurses Phase II (Source: Nurses 24 units, n=718) %
Regional	40.53	40.95
Sub-regional	29.05	27.16
District	30.42	31.89

Table 2.4a · Functional and clinical grades of study **responders** (% of total grade/title recruited)

Title	Grade A	B	C	D	E	F	G	H	I	TOT	% recruited
CNM								4	8	12	80.0
CNS							1	14	2	17	100
CNT								7	1	8	88.9
SR						62	127			189	84.4
SM					76	33				109	85.8
SN				15	108	29				152	75.6
C405				6	21	8	1			36	70.6
EN			11	28	5					44	71.0
NN		31	45							76	71.7
NAux	15	4								19	63.3
Bank		6	7	17	23	3				56	69.1
Total	15	41	63	66	233	135	129	25	11	718	
% recruited	60.0	69.5	75.9	66.7	76.4	82.8	87.2	86.2	91.7		

A further small group of parents whose babies died were recruited from the same units and participated in the study, returning specifically designed questionnaires relating to their situation: a total of 19 were initially approached by letter, 14 responded positively (74%) and 12 (60%) returned completed questionnaires. Their data, apart from that on birthweight, gestational age and reasons for admission, are presented separately in the chapter on parents and neonatal care.

Additional Data Collection

Further data collection similar to that undertaken in Phase I was carried out in 1994 with 24 neonatal units (six regional units, six subregional units and twelve

Table 2.4b · Functional and clinical grades of study **non-responders** (% of total grade or title recruited)

Title	Grade A	B	C	D	E	F	G	H	I	TOT	% recruited
CNM								2	1	3	20.0
CNS											
CNT								1		1	11.1
SR						15	19	1		35	15.6
SM					15	3				18	14.2
SN				11	29	9				49	24.4
C405				2	12	1				15	29.4
EN			3	11	4					18	29.0
NN		14	14	2						30	28.3
NAux	10		1							11	36.7
Bank		4	2	7	12					25	30.9
Total	10	18	20	33	72	28	19	4	1	205	
% recruited	40.0	30.5	24.1	33.3	23.6	17.2	12.8	13.8	8.3		

Key to Table 2.4

CNM = Clinical Nurse Manager
CNS = Clinical Nurse Specialist
CNT = Clinical Nurse Teacher
SR   = Sister
SM   = Staff Midwife
SN   = Staff Nurse

C405 = ENB course 405 student
EN   = Enrolled Nurse
NN   = Nursery Nurse
NAux = Nursing Auxiliary
Bank = Reserve nursing staff

district units). Details of medical and nurse staffing were collected and used to compare with data from the main study.

Data Analysis

Following data entry and checking, the study data were analysed using the Statistical Package for the Social Sciences (SPSS/PC+ Version 4.0). For many of the largely descriptive data no statistical tests were necessary. Where questions concerned differences between groups, the appropriate chi-square test was used. Where the relationship between two groups and an ordinal variable was being examined a Mann-Witney U test was performed and when larger numbers of groups were compared a Kruskal Wallis test was used. Where the relationship between two ordinal variables was in question, a correlation coefficient was calculated. Spearman's rank correlation was used unless both variables could be assumed to be normally distributed, in which case Pearson's r was calculated. Correlations and significance levels are given in the text as appropriate. Multivariate analyses were carried out on the individual nurse data and details of these are given in the text in Chapter 8.

The Research Findings

The results of the study are introduced, presented and discussed separately in seven chapters covering the main areas addressed by the research. The earlier chapters centre on the general areas of organisation and staffing, nursing skill mix, training and education and the changing role of the nurse in neonatal care. Those that come later focus more on individual factors and the personal circumstances of those working in the specialty. Thus the later chapters are on the position of neonatal nurses as working women, their physical health and psychological wellbeing and the views and experiences of parents whose babies are cared for in neonatal units. The final chapter consists of a short discussion concerning the implications of the research findings and refers both to future research and the wider context of health care provision. An executive summary follows containing a synopsis of the results and recommendations.

Throughout the chapters detailing the research findings the words of nurses, doctors and parents are used to illustrate and illuminate the points being made. The quotations, with slight modifications to prevent individual identification and maintain confidentiality, come directly from the replies the subjects themselves wrote in responding to open-ended sections of the questionnaires.

References

Bortner, R. W. and Rosenman, R. H. (1967) The measurement of Pattern A behaviour. *Journal of Chronic Diseases*, **20**, 525–533.

Department of Health. (1989) Survey of Nurses in High Technology Care. NHS Management Executive. London.

Department of Health (1991) Local Research Ethics Committees. HSG(91)5, August. DOH, London.

Goldberg, D. and Williams, P. (1988) A User's Guide to the General Health Questionnaire. NFER-Nelson, Windsor, Berkshire.

Harris, P., Hingley, P. and Cooper, C. (1988) Nurse Stress Index. Resource Assessment, Harrogate.

Hingley, P., and Cooper, C. (1986) Stress and the Nurse Manager. Wiley, Chichester.

Neuberger, J. (1992) Ethics and Health Care: The Role of Research Ethics Committees in the United Kingdom. Research Report no. 13, Kings Fund, London.

The Royal College of Physicians. (1988) Medical Care of The Newborn in England and Wales. RCP, London.

Spelton, E. R., Smith, I., Totterdell, P. A. I., Barton, J., Folkard, S. and Bohle, P. (1993) The relationship between coping strategies and GHQ scores in nurses. *Ergonomics*, **36**, 227–232.

Chapter 3 · Organisation and Staffing

Organisational Issues

The aim in this part of the study was to explore some of the critical issues concerning the current organisation and management of neonatal care. Similarities and differences between units are used to illustrate the degree to which consensus and conformity was evident in staffing numbers and structures.

Many different factors influence what happens in neonatal units. The fundamental elements that underlie the wellbeing and welfare of patients and staff are considered in this chapter. These are the status and capacity of the units, that is the numbers of cots available for sick or small newborns, and the capability, that is the structure and numbers of nursing and medical personnel used and required to run the service. Other factors include the proximity to other hospitals and the organisation of specialist services at a regional and super-regional level.

Nurse Staffing Levels

Excessive workload and understaffing are potential stressors in all occupations and many previous studies have identified these as among the most important stress factors for health-care professionals (Gray-Toft and Anderson, 1981; Hingley and Cooper, 1986). For individual nurses, senior and junior, working in small and large neonatal units, the staffing levels are a prime concern and a central issue in their everyday working lives.

> 'I was looking after sixteen babies with only one junior and one bank nurse. Eleven of the babies were high dependency and I was trying to supervise the other nurses and deal with new admissions, one of which was a baby whose father was completely distraught. I had no time, even to say hello to him'

> 'On a recent shift I had to look after two ventilated and two high dependency babies, all unstable. I felt that they did not receive the care they deserved and frustrated at having to give less than I am capable of'.

> 'The workload varies enormously from one shift to the next. Staffing is adequate for some shifts, but sickness and admissions can stretch the staff beyond acceptable limits.'

'When there are plenty of staff you have fewer babies to look after, and at the end of the day you feel that you have looked after your babies properly.'

Nurse Staffing Models

It is generally agreed that the nursing establishment set, traditionally measured in Whole Time Equivalents (WTEs) should relate to the type of unit, the kind of babies cared for, the number of cots and the facilities available (Walker, 1983).

A range of methods have been used to calculate nurse staffing needs (Jones et al, 1993a; Arthur and James,1994). These largely fall into three types of approach: consensus, "top-down" and "bottom-up" methods. The use of a "top down" method for calculating staffing requirements based on the recommendations of the professional organisations involved in neonatal care, though open to debate, enables comparisons to be made between a large number of units and at different points in time. Individual units can also compare their own staffing levels directly with those of other units in the region or nationally.

"Bottom up" activity and workload analyses are not practicable on a large scale and are not at this time a satisfactory or manageable alternative for most NHS hospital trusts. The methodology and sampling framework is critical in work activity studies and many are undertaken over too short a time period to encompass the variations in workload normally encountered. However, as a means of validating "top down" methods and assisting in their revision, they can be useful. Due to local differences in organisation and policy, the generalisability of locally based studies like those of the Northern Neonatal Network (1994) or Williams et al (1994), is doubtful as the authors themselves emphasise. Hospital or unit information systems where they are in operation and accessible could be invaluable. With data recorded on admissions, occupancy and case-mix, in conjunction with workload studies, they can be used as an audit tool to inform local organisational and staffing issues. However, problems of comparability can arise with different information systems and the extent to which such systems are in operation continues to vary between and within trusts (Jones et al, 1993a).

The method of assessment and comparison in this study involved a "top-down" method of calculating and contrasting the nursing needs in the neonatal unit. Details of the numbers of staff employed, the current establishment and numbers of intensive and special care cots were obtained in Phase I. Using these data on the 56 study units several hypothetical staffing models were examined and the degree to which each unit fitted these was calculated. The models are based on the staffing guidelines given in the Sheldon Report (1971) and reiterated in the Court Report (1976), the Report by the Standing Joint Committee of the British Paediatric Association and the Royal College of Obstetrics and Gynaecology (1983), the Royal College of Physicians report (1988) and a circular from the British Paediatric Association and the British Association for Perinatal Medicine (1992). These are summarised below in Table 3.1.

Using the Sheldon 1971 recommendations, a theoretical model of nurse staffing in relation to cots is shown (Figure 3.1). Utilising this model, the levels of over or understaffing in operation in the study units at the end of 1990 are shown (Figure 3.2). Similar models, based on higher nursing staff to patient ratios, show increasingly steeper slopes as the numbers of nurses per baby per 24 hours is increased. The BPA and RCOG (1983) recommendations were used for a second model (Figure 3.3) and the RCP (1988) for a third model (Figure 3.4).

The extent to which the neonatal nursing establishments fell above or below the level recommended using the different criteria is shown. Using Model 1, in 1990 thirteen study units fell below the levels recommended in 1971. These were one regional centre, two sub-regional centres and ten district units. The proportion by which the individual units fell below the recommendation ranged from 1% to 54%. (Two units scoring 0, being at exactly the set level were assigned either side of the zero for the purposes of the figure and are not included in the thirteen referred to above).

Using Model 2 more than half the units in the study (31) fell below the establishment recommended in 1983. These were nearly half the regional units in the study, more than three-quarters of the sub-regional units and half of the district units studied. The proportion by which the individual units fell below the recommendation ranged from 3% to 63%.

Using Model 3 only four of the fifty-six units in the study reached the level of five nurses per intensive care cot and 1.5 per special care cot as recommended in 1988. These were one regional centre and three district units. The most recent recommendations in which a "high dependency" category was introduced (1992) are also listed in Table 3.1. Some units used this term to describe babies, but most did not designate cots in this way. However, among the few units for which data are available, there was wide variation: one regional centre was within 2% of the recommended level of staffing while another was 59% below.

In general, it seems that no common policy is in operation nationally, though senior hospital staff commonly said they were working towards what had been recommended by the English National Board for Nursing Midwifery and Health Visiting (1987, 1991). Units of a particular type were no more likely to be appropriately staffed according to any of the different criteria and associated models. As in nursing more generally, inequalities of the kind described seem to be reflecting historic patterns of resource allocation rather than differences in case-mix (Jones et al, 1993b). With regard to the question of understaffing or overstaffing, this obviously depends on the model or standard adopted. On the first and earliest model, a large proportion of neonatal units, but not all, could be considered as overstaffed in nursing establishment terms. In contrast, very few units reached the levels set in the third model and more than two-thirds could be considered markedly understaffed.

Table 3.1 · Successive recommendations for neonatal unit staffing

	Qualified Nursing Staff Required Over a 24 hour period	
	Per Intensive Care Cot	Per Special Care Cot
Sheldon (1971) (MODEL 1)	3	1
BPA and RCOG (1983) (MODEL 2)	4	1.25
ENB (1987) *Minimum*	4	1.25
Optimum	5	1.5
RCP (1988) (MODEL 3)	5	1.5
BPA, BAPM, NNA (1992)	5.5 + 3.5 per High Dependency Cot	1

3 STAFF PER IC COT, 1 PER SC COT

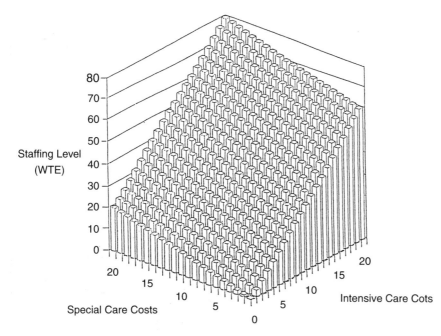

Figure 3.1 · Theoretical nursing establishment model 1 showing numbers of staff required

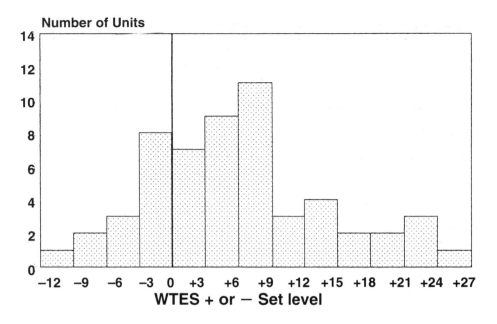

Figure 3.2 · Establishment match with model 1 (3 nurses per intensive care cot, 1 per special care cot) n=56 units

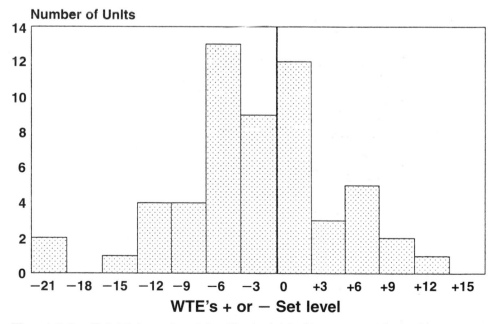

Figure 3.3 · Establishment match with model 2, (4 nurses per intensive care cot, 1.25 per special care cot) n=56 units

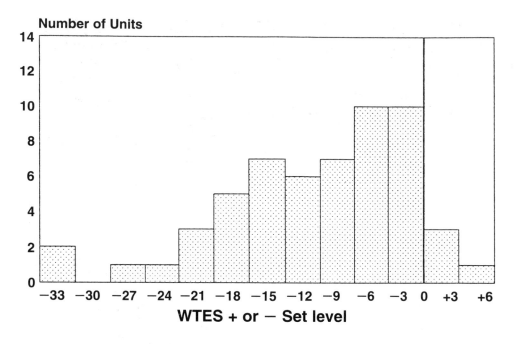

Figure 3.4 · Establishment match with model 3, (5 nurses per intensive care cot, 1.5 per special care cot) n=56 units

Nurse Staffing Update

Large inter-unit variation and understaffing continues to occur. Using recent data collected on 24 units shows that in 1994, using Model 2, more than half the establishments were less than what had been recommended ten years previously: 12 of the 24 were more than 10% below the 1984 recommendation. These were two regional, four subregional and six district units. The proportion by which the units fell below the ratio of 4 WTE nurses per intensive care cot and 1.25 per special care cot varied between 41% and 1%.

As previously, very few units (2 out of 24) were positive using Model 3. Calculating the match or mismatch based on the more recent recommendations (BPA/NNA, 1992) showed that where high dependency cots were designated (11 out of the 24 units), the average discrepancy in 1994 was 28% below the requirement. Where only intensive and special care cots were designated, the mean difference was 9% less than required. By including high dependency in the special care category this is likely to have resulted in an underestimation of the staffing need in these units.

A comparison of the distribution of 56 units in 1990 and 24 units in 1994 (using Model 2 and the 1984 recommendation) shows that though the range in discrepancy is smaller, with a smaller proportion of units being at the extremes of under-staffing, there was no significant difference between 1990 and the present.

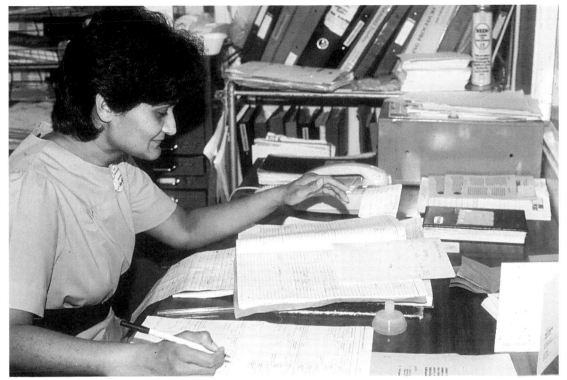

Sister in charge arranging staffing and cover for the neonatal unit

Responses to a Shortfall

The strategies that can be utilised in coping with a shortfall in staffing numbers and the service implications of these are shown in Figure 3.5. Formal establishment reviews are not carried out at regular intervals and are often a response to a crisis. Some appear to be undertaken reluctantly, while others are part of a "skill-mix review". Other measures and possible responses to staff shortages are limited: present staff can be used for longer or additional shifts; overlap times and break allowances can be reduced; bank or agency staff can be employed; staff can be lent by other departments, or those on duty are simply expected to cope. All of these strategies were recorded amongst the units studied:

'I was on annual leave, but the unit was so short-staffed I was telephoned three times and asked to come in and work.'

'Almost every shift I have to spend a great deal of time trying to bring in bank or agency staff, to bring the staffing levels up to the minimum'

'Our district hospital has no officially designated intensive care cots, and I was in charge, with one enrolled nurse, one staff nurse

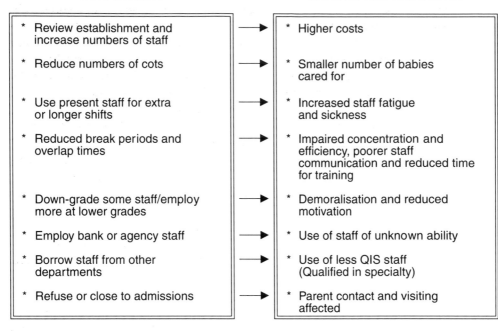

STRATEGIES	SERVICE IMPLICATIONS
* Review establishment and increase numbers of staff	* Higher costs
* Reduce numbers of cots	* Smaller number of babies cared for
* Use present staff for extra or longer shifts	* Increased staff fatigue and sickness
* Reduced break periods and overlap times	* Impaired concentration and efficiency, poorer staff communication and reduced time for training
* Down-grade some staff/employ more at lower grades	* Demoralisation and reduced motivation
* Employ bank or agency staff	* Use of staff of unknown ability
* Borrow staff from other departments	* Use of less QIS staff (Qualified in specialty)
* Refuse or close to admissions	* Parent contact and visiting affected

Figure 3.5 · Possible responses to a shortfall in neonatal unit staffing in terms of organisational strategies and service implications

borrowed from the postnatal ward, and an agency nurse to care for 13 babies, including a sick ventilated baby and another who was severely asphyxiated and terminally ill.'

'You are expected to work your days off and made to feel guilty if you say no. We are always being phoned to work extra duties when at home or on holiday.'

'On a late shift at a weekend the unit was very busy and not safely staffed. The sister in charge contacted the manager, but no extra help was given. Staff are regularly expected to provide safe nursing care under tremendous pressure'

Of the 718 individual nurses participating in the second phase of the study, 47% had worked extra shifts in the previous twelve months to cover staff shortages and 40% had worked long or split shifts (Figure 3.6). The regional units were more likely to have asked staff to do extra shifts, while in the smaller units nurses more often worked longer or split shifts. Of the nurses surveyed, 89% were employed with a permanent contract, but 8% were regularly employed as bank or agency staff. A further 3% were learners, caring for babies while on a neonatal course (ENB 405, 409).

Overlap time is used for handover from one shift to another and as a time when staff are available for teaching sessions, ward rounds and meetings. The extent of effective utilization of overlap has been questioned (Audit Commission, 1991; Hawley and Stilwell, 1993), though not in the area of neonatal care. As a measure directed at financial savings, shift overlap time has been shortened or cut in some units, thus eroding the time that can be used in this way. Among the 56 study units, details of the overlap time was as follows: for the early shift it ranged from 15 minutes to 4 hours (mean 2 hours 41 minutes); for the late shift the range was from no time at all to 90 minutes (mean 26 minutes); for the night shift it was from nothing to 1 hour 45 minutes (mean 24 minutes). Shortening or abandoning overlap time all together reduces staff hours and immediate financial costs (Audit Commission, 1993), but may have adverse effects on both effective handover, care and discharge planning and the availability of opportunities for continuing education and update.

The quality and duration of handover can vary depending on the organisation of nursing care. Most of the units were using a nursing process model of care (48 of the 56) and only two were using a primary nursing model. Direct allocation of babies has made handover more effective for those patients, but not of the unit as a whole. Working in nursing teams, with a group of nurses directly assigned to a group of patients, as occurs with team nursing, aims to facilitate the exchange of information and continuity of care. However, it seems that relatively few units (6 out of 56) were actually working in this way.

From an individual perspective and from the management point of view, staffing levels are a highly salient issue. At the time of the study, nursing staff in many units were looking after more babies and more intensive care babies than

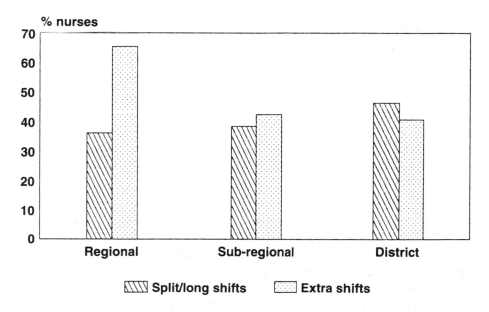

Figure 3.6 · Additional cover provided by nurses during the previous twelve months (n=24 units, 718 nurses)

Sheldon or any of the professional bodies or advisory groups have recommended. On their last shift, some staff nurses and staff midwives had directly looked after as many as five babies needing intensive care:

> 'I was allocated five ICU babies on a late shift because of short staffing. I could not leave the room I was working in and did not get a proper break throughout the 7½ hour shift. I had to supervise parents, give IV drugs, nurse ventilated babies and change long lines as well as other general tasks – I felt that I was chasing my tail and not carrying out my job properly.'

Though this was relatively uncommon, looking after two or three intensive care babies, as well as others less seriously ill, was frequent and continues to occur.

The Provision of Neonatal Cots

As was discussed in the previous section, nurse staffing levels are calculated on the basis of the numbers of cots that a unit has to staff, equip and maintain. The fluctuations in workload that are common in this area make the planning and organisation of neonatal services difficult. On the ground the problems are evident:

> 'I came on duty to find 30 babies in 24 cot spaces, one preterm baby was expected and unbooked twenty-five week twins were about to be delivered. Enter three new babies: no space, no equipment and insufficient nursing staff'

> 'We were really busy, the unit was officially closed, but babies still kept arriving. There was not enough equipment, and what we had kept failing. We were short of staff and there were eight babies in an area designated for five. There was no time between observations and feeding for anything but basic nursing care'

> 'The unit is always busy and we often turn babies away. I feel there should be more awareness of the critical situation neonatal units are in."

The Sheldon Report (1971), in addition to making recommendations about staffing levels, also sought to advise on the numbers of neonatal cots. The provision of six cots per 1000 live births was put forward as a guideline to be used in planning neonatal services. Included within this figure was one cot per 1000 live births designated for intensive care. The Report of the Royal College of Physicians (1988), while recommending the same over-all figure for cots, suggested that of the six cots provided 1.5 should be allocated for intensive care and 4.5 for special care.

The data collected from 56 study hospitals on the total live births for 1989 and the total numbers of designated special and intensive care cots in 1990, were used to examine the degree to which the Sheldon (1971) recommendations were in operation in the study units across the country. Figure 3.7 shows the number of units that met the criteria for the numbers of designated cots and the extent of the match or mismatch. As with nurse staffing levels, the inter-unit variation was marked. Comparing hospitals using the figure for live births in 1989 shows large differences: seventeen of the 56 (30%) were more than three cots below the requirement and seven (13%) more than three cots above. However, the majority of those units that had well over the numbers of cots calculated as necessary for their inborn population were regional units which admit babies from over a large area.

Management information returned in Phase I indicated that at times 34 of the 56 units (61%) admitted babies requiring intensive care, for whom no designated cots were available. (These were 9 of the 14 regional units studied, 9 of the 14 subregional units and 16 of the 28 district units.) Fewer units (27%) admitted babies requiring special care without the cots actually being available, though this was not uncommon (4 regional units, 6 subregional units and 5 district units). These data may underestimate the extent to which, in the present situation, many units are more commonly accepting additional babies when they are already technically "full".

The recommendation regarding the provision of intensive and special care cots is a general one, however, the need for cots may vary by region according to the live births. In the RCP report (1988), a theoretical figure for intensive care cots was derived for each of the health regions, based on numbers of live births and an assumed cot occupancy of 70%. The figure thus calculated ranged from 1.27 in Wessex to 1.59 in North Western. Whether these or similar figures have been used in actually designating cots in different regions is unclear. More recently, findings from a Northern Neonatal Network (1993b) study carried

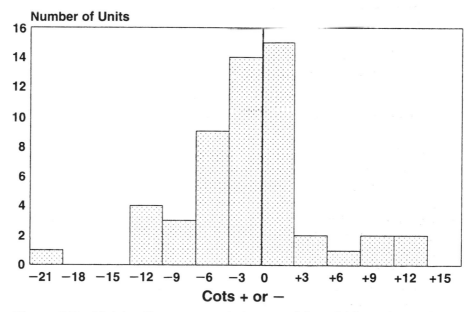

Figure 3.7 · Match with recommended cot provision of 1 intensive and 5 special care cots per 1000 live births (n=56)

out in 1991 show that in one region at least, the need for high dependency cots (including intensive care) is lower than this and is in the region of one per thousand live births. Concentrating long-term high dependency and intensive care in a small number of units (five in total) and working in a collaborative way is put forward as an effective means of organising this aspect of neonatal care.

Using the Sheldon recommendation and linking the number of cots to births shows an under-provision of cots and, like nurse staffing numbers, provides further evidence of marked inter-unit variation. However, general recommendations can seem far from the day-to-day fluctuations in the numbers of babies needing care: differences between regions and changing patterns of care, for example the inclusion of a transitional care element, complicate the issue further. The under-provision of cots in some of the study units reported here may indicate a real discrepancy or may be a consequence of an over-generous formula. Fluctuations in the annual number of births occur and it would have been preferable to use live birth data for a number of years, rather than just 1989 in the calculations. However, as the data were analysed for each unit separately, this is unlikely to have altered the finding substantially.

The kind of problems described so graphically continue to arise:

> 'I was helping to admit a 32 week BBA baby to intensive care in a room with a terminally ill baby being specialled on a day when we had new doctors and registrar starting and not enough staff to help and cope with the situation. It was 07.30 hrs and a very stressful way to start the day – which didn't get any better. I also had babies of my own to look after in another room.'

> 'I was working in intensive care with one other member of staff. 28 babies in total were on the unit, with just five staff: 1 G grade, 3 D's and 1 E.'

Further data collected in 1994 on cots show that though the majority of units appear to have maintained the same number of cots, some have reduced their numbers, most commonly in the special care category. Others have increased or are planning to increase the numbers of intensive care and high dependency cots they provide.

Somehow, in managing the service, it seems that workload variations must be taken into account and the maximum number of sick babies that can be cared for at any one time included in the provision calculations. The idea that neonatal units have "elastic walls" and "ever-open doors" and that the staff are able to "take on whatever is thrown at us", is one that founders in the face of the realities of complex high technology care:

> 'The consultant admitted some out of area babies who required intensive care, which meant that all the babies only received minimal levels of care because of the shortage of skilled staff.'

> 'When asked to admit a baby from another unit we were already over full and had the possibility of more preterm admissions. There

was a lot of staff sickness and we had to borrow equipment as there were more patients than we were funded for. On requesting transfer of the baby to another unit equally well equipped and able to deal with the problem, the reply from the medical staff was that no baby could be transferred out and we would have to "muddle through".'

What ever the method of calculation, the levels of staffing and cot provision have implications for nursing and medical staff, and babies and their families.

'I was in total charge of the unit and looking after seven low dependency babies. Junior staff did not get my help or support. Obstetric and paediatric staff were unable to accept that we were full, resulting in a lack of support, lack of good care and unnecessary arguments.'

"The unit has had a high number of intensive care and special care babies, with insufficient staff. So everyone has been working just to do the job, not obtaining any job satisfaction."

Matching service provision to a variable need is a problem inherent in many areas of acute care. Flexible mechanisms are required that can work across trust boundaries as well as evidence-based structuring of the service. When cots are not available and babies have to be transferred some distance, or when units are full and still more babies are accepted, the consequences may be profound. (Parents' experiences of transfer are discussed in Chapter 9.)

Nursing Staff Turnover and Vacancies

The data that were used to examine the three different models of nurse staffing are based on full establishments. However, with staff changes, and in some instances as a matter of policy, some units were being run at a lower level than the one set. Thus the extent of mismatch with the models discussed above would actually have been greater had these nursing vacancies been taken into account.

Data on the extent to which establishments were not filled were collected for all the study units in Phase I. Across all the units the proportion of the nursing establishment that was vacant at the time of the study was 8% (145 vacant WTEs out of a total of 1753 WTEs). This was less than was found in the Survey of Nurses in High Technology Care (DOH, 1989), where a rate of 12.4% was reported. For the different types of unit there was a significant difference in the proportion of the establishment that was vacant ($p=<0.05$), being highest for the regional centres at 10%, followed by the subregional units (9%) and then the district units (6%).

Data collected on 24 units in 1994 show a larger proportion of units with no vacancies and an over all rate of 6% (53 vacant WTEs out of a total of 891 WTEs). A significant difference between the differently sized units was not found with this smaller number of units, where the rates were 7% for regional and district units and 4% for the subregional units. In terms of the vacancies (in WTEs) in 1990 the majority of these (52%) were in regional units, all of which were located in teaching hospitals. Fewer were in subregional units (29%) and in district units (19%). Data from 1994 also show the majority of vacancies (49%) to be in regional centres, with relatively fewer in subregional units (16%) and more (35%) in district units.

The overall turnover rate for NHS staff reported for a study carried out at approximately the same time as the present one (Gray and Phillips, 1994) was 13.6%. Turnover was found to be higher amongst non-nursing staff, however, the rate for registered nurses and health visitors at 14.1% was slightly higher than that reported for midwives (11.1%). No breakdown of the rates by specialty, title, or type of hospital was available that could be used for comparison with the present study. Turnover of neonatal nursing staff was calculated using the total number of nurses leaving permanently during the whole of 1989 as a proportion of the total number of nurses employed by grade at the time of the study. Using this method, the nursing staff turnover rate across all the study units was found to be slightly higher at 16% than the rates referred to above. It was also significantly different according to the type of unit ($p=<0.01$), with regional centres having a turnover of 22%, subregional units 14% and district units a rate of 9%.

The introduction of new members of staff can present an opportunity to inject new skills, interest and enthusiasm into a unit. However, when valued and experienced members of staff leave for another unit or a change of specialty, the effects on morale, motivation and efficiency may be marked, especially if they are not replaced by staff at a similar level:

'Staff change so often, you just get them trained and used to your ways of doing things and then off they go!'

'Nine experienced members of staff have resigned over a short period and have only been replaced by newly-qualified RGNs and inexperienced staff nurses, increasing the workload for those who have stayed,'

'In the three years that I have worked on the unit, there has been a very high turnover of staff who all seem to leave for similar reasons – discontentment, disillusionment, lack of promotion, broken promises, feeling used, problems with off-duty. The management have made no changes or even attempts to understand the problems, to the detriment of the whole unit.'

'As a new member of staff I was expected to take responsibility for intensive care babies without supervision and support during my first week on the unit and since then. I had no previous experience in this area, except my midwifery training several years before.'

'Newly qualified nurses, with no midwifery or neonatal experience are now being employed and we have to teach and supervise them as well as doing our usual routine and other work.'

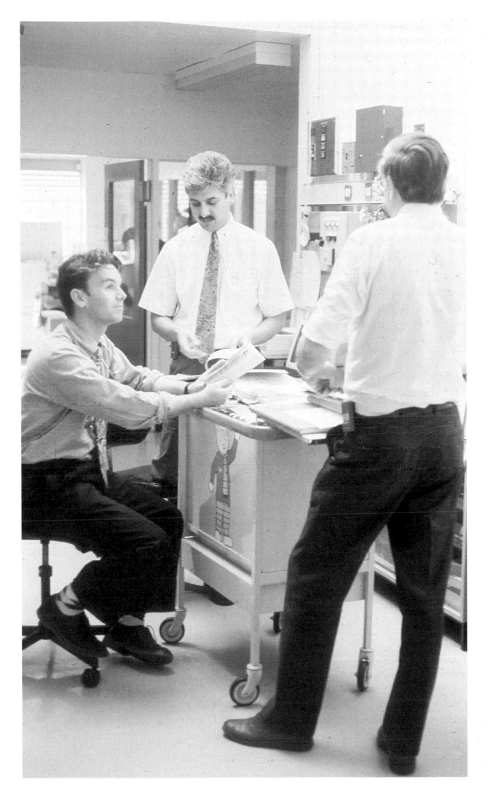

Consultant, senior registrar and house officer discussing NICU patients at a ward round

A wide range of reasons were given for leaving posts in neonatal nursing, many of which related to further training and advancement. Factors relating to post-basic education and career development will be discussed in Chapter 5 on training and education and Chapter 7 on neonatal nurses as working women.

Medical Staffing in Neonatal Care

The numbers, experience, background and training of medical staff and the way that medical cover is organised are vitally important aspects of neonatal care that have significant implications for nurses working in the specialty. The structure and organisation of the medical team affects many aspects of neonatal nursing, including the overall quality of care and the way that it is delivered. The extent to which medical staff are qualified, experienced, motivated and available contributes to produce very different working environments. Where medical staff work long hours on unsatisfactory on-call rotas, and where there are demanding clinical responsibilities in other departments, sometimes on separate sites, the burden is likely to be increased for nursing staff.

Doctor Numbers

Information about the medical staffing and cover was obtained for the 56 study units on a total of 416 doctors. The relative proportions of the different grades of medical staff working in the different types of neonatal unit are shown in Figure 3.8. In order to give a picture of the actual numbers of staff employed at the different levels, the mean numbers of the staff employed in each type of unit are shown in Figure 3.9.

Some variation was evident in the medical staff working in the different types of neonatal unit. One or more neonatologists (paediatricians experienced and accredited in neonatal medicine) were working in all but one of the regional centres, though in only two of the fourteen centres were there the three medical staff recommended at this level (RCP, 1988). Neonatologists were not employed in ten of the fourteen sub-regional units, nor were there any in the twenty-eight district units in the study. Variation was also found in the employment of middle-grade medical staff. All but one of the regional units studied had at least one registrar and one senior registrar, though only four of the sub-regional units had both. None of these large centres had the four registrar-level staff recommended (RCP, 1988) and the majority of sub-regional units had only registrars. Differences also occurred among the district units: of the twenty-eight in the study, two had a senior registrar and a registrar; two had only a senior registrar, and seven had neither.

Senior House Officers (SHOs) carry out much of the routine clinical work in neonatal units. The number of SHOs working in any unit varied with the type and size, but not systematically. For example, the number employed in regional centres ranged from 2 to 6 dedicated SHOs. Where the number employed in these large units was low, this appeared, in some instances, to be balanced by the presence of more middle-grade medical staff. In smaller units senior

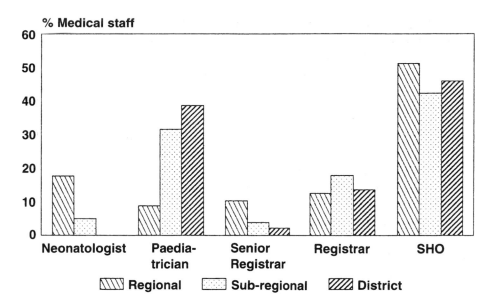

Figure 3.8 · Medical staff employed at different grades in different types of neonatal unit (n=56 units)

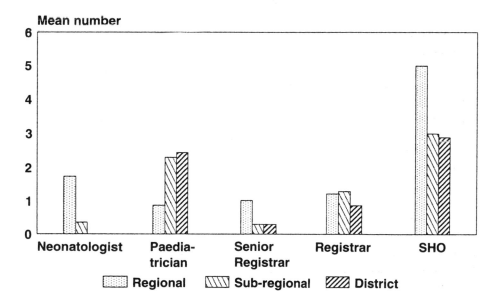

Figure 3.9 · Mean number of medical staff employed at different grades in different types of unit (n=56 units)

medical staff expressed concern about both the experience and turnover of junior doctors:

> 'The safety net is inadequate on two nights out of three, when an inexperienced SHO is 1st on call. We badly need more experienced SHOs and a registrar.'

> 'The experience of junior staff is limited. After a short period of 2–3 weeks, they usually pick up intubation skills. But after 3 months they move to general paediatrics, and start another induction period.'

> 'I don't think GP trainees should be working in neonatal care at all. They don't need this kind of experience and most find it extremely stressful.'

The proportion of junior medical staff with previous paediatric or neonatal experience varied significantly with unit type (p=<0.001): 66% for SHOs working in regional units, 28% for subregional units and 21% for district units. Accurate information about the numbers of non-consultant medical staff "dedicated" to neonatal care was not available from all the questionnaire returns, though these were more likely to be recorded as present in the larger units, most commonly the regional centres.

Cover Arrangements

The on-call cover situation reported for units of different type is illustrated in Figure 3.10. In all units on-call cover was provided by a consultant and where there were registrars and senior registrars they participated in the rota. For consultants in 31 of the 56 units (55%) the on-call rota at this time was a 1 in 3, though in 16 (29%) they were working a 1 in 2 rota. The latter was almost as common in large as smaller units (3 out of 14 regional units, 3 out of 14 subregional units and 10 out of 28 district units).

For units with senior registrars (21 out of 56) and units with registrars (46 out of 56) the most frequent cover arrangement was also a 1 in 3 (49% of units with senior registrar staff and 72% of units with registrar level staff). In 70% of units (40 out of 56) SHOs also covered on a 1 in 3 basis. In only 14% of units (8) was a day and night shift system in operation and that was most likely for SHOs in regional centres (5 out of 14).

Thus most of the regional centres had "adequate" cover at consultant and registrar level and the situation was to some extent similar for sub-regional units. The situation for district units, on the other hand was less flexible and at this time they were largely dependent on consultant cover only:

> 'We are restricted in employing essential middle grade staff. We also need another consultant with an interest in neonatal paediatrics.'

> 'We have a 3 in 1 rota and insufficient consultant time, but the main problem is split-site working.'

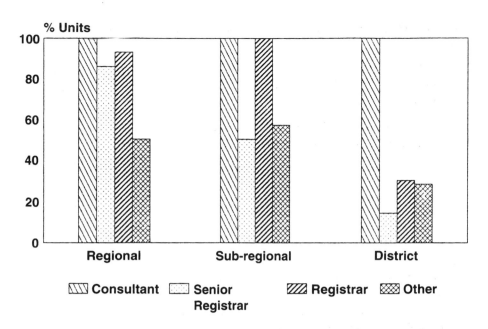

Figure 3.10 · On-call cover by medical staff other than SHOs for different types of neonatal unit (n=56 units)

'We are all very thinly spread. The district serves a large area. Out-patient sessions are held on a site remote from SCBU. Other clinics are held further away. All paediatric consultants have heavy commitments outside SCBU and the SHOs on call have to move between two different sites 4 miles apart.'

Medical Responsibilities Outside Neonatal care

The extent to which medical staff working in neonatal units have responsibilities in paediatric and other departments can affect the way in which their work is organised, but also has consequences for neonatal nursing staff and patients.

The on-call responsibilities in other departments for different types of staff and in the three types of unit are illustrated in Figure 3.11. Among all three types of unit there was some commitment to cover other departments, usually paediatrics and accident and emergency. This appeared to be greatest for the sub-regional and district units, where at times the medical staff on duty were needed in two places at the same time. On-call responsibilities of this kind were most frequent for consultants in the sub-regional units (13 out of 14) and district units (26 out of 28), registrars in the sub-regional units (13 out of 14) and SHOs in the district units (24 out of 28).

If staff can be called to work in other departments outside the unit, then it was felt that the proximity or otherwise of these must be considered. Split

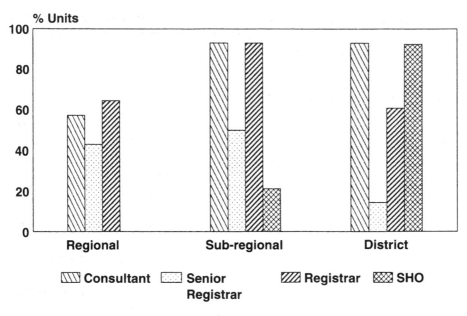

Figure 3.11 · On call responsibilities for unit medical staff in paediatric and A & E departments (n=56 units)

hospital sites or widely separated buildings can exacerbate the problems of organising and coordinating care. Data were collected on the location of the study units in relation to other facilities. Of the 56 delivery suites 38 (68%) were on the same floor as the neonatal unit, but 18 (32%) were on a different floor or further away. Some paediatric wards (19) were in the same building (34%), but the rest were either on the same (22, 39%) or another site (7, 14%), or even at a different hospital all together (8, 13%). Many Accident and Emergency departments were in the same building or on the same site (33, 59%), though a substantial number were located on another site (8, 14%) or at another hospital (15, 27%). Not all these departments in all these locations were covered by staff from neonatal care, but many units clearly assisted in providing emergency cover in a number of separate locations.

In some hospitals the relationship between paediatric departments and neonatal units is closer than one based simply on cover. A small number of units were moving in the direction of integrating paediatric and neonatal intensive care, a process not without its attendant problems. In other units the relationship is a formal, if limited one.

> 'Because there are no facilities for ventilation on the paediatric ward, non-neonates are admitted or readmitted for intensive or post-operative care to SCBU.'

The admission of non-neonates, that is of older children who are very seriously ill, to the neonatal unit puts additional pressures on both medical and nursing staff. Of the 24 units visited 19 (79%) admitted non-neonates. Recent admissions had included suspected meningitis, respiratory syncytial virus, and non-accidental injury. Such arrangements can occur where facilities and staffing arrangements are less than adequate.

Update on Medical Staffing and Cover

The data collected on this aspect of neonatal unit organisation in 1994 show that there have been some changes in medical staffing, probably as a result of the various initiatives in this area (Higginson, 1992; DOH, 1993). Greater numbers of neonatologists and consultants with a special interest in neonatal care have been employed in senior posts. Relatively greater numbers of middle grade staff have also been employed; only 2 of 24 units in 1994 had no staff at registrar level and more than half had staff in registrar and senior registrar posts.

Relatively greater numbers of SHOs have been employed, though the degree to which those in post in 1994 had previous experience differed little from that found in 1990. A total of 36% (43 out of 118 SHOs working in 24 neonatal units) compared with 38% in 1990, had previous experience in paediatrics or neonatal care. More than a third of all SHOs employed were working as GP trainees, all of whom were located in subregional or district units, representing 46% and 53% of staff at SHO level respectively in these types of unit.

Based on recent evidence, the on-call cover situation appears to have improved since 1990 in line with changes brought about by the Department of Health directives and the working of the regional taskforces. The most common rotas for consultants working in neonatal care are 1 in 3 (42%) or 1 in 4 (42%). A similar situation exists at registrar level. More shift systems have been introduced and day and night or partial shifts for SHOs are in operation in 54% of units (13 out of 24), though this was significantly less likely in district units (p=<0.01).

Thus with greater numbers of medical staff at all levels, the better cover arrangements reported, less onerous rotas for senior and junior medical staff and the introduction of partial and day and night shifts for the latter, the medical staffing situation seems to have improved markedly. The problems with split sites and widely separated departments for which medical staff have responsibilities still occur, though as staff numbers are increased, these are less acute.

What's in a Number?

The deficits in paediatric intensive care staffing and provision, and the shortfall in beds and nurses qualified in the specialty, have been well documented in a British Paediatric Association report (1993) and find echoes among the data presented here. However, it is of interest that with patients who also need intensive or high dependency care, the staffing levels recommended are higher (6.4 WTEs per open bed) than those put forward for neonatal intensive care.

This difference has not gone unnoticed among neonatal nurses who feel that though their patients may be smaller, "the need for nursing care is just the same".

As was found with paediatric intensive care, this study of neonatal care showed large inter-unit variation in the levels of medical and nurse staffing. The nursing establishments set, cots provided and medical staffing arrangements were found to be at lower levels in many units than those recommended by professional and other bodies. The relationship between the nursing establishment and the numbers of designated intensive and special care cots in each unit was examined using different models of staffing based on successive recommendations. The more recent the recommendation, the greater the discrepancy between the theoretical establishment set by the institution and establishment and that recommended.

If the nursing establishment actually in operation is considered and nursing vacancies taken into account, the discrepancies are further enlarged. There were also instances in which local factors operated to produce anomalies: in one unit a staff nurse permanently employed on a paediatric ward was officially listed on the neonatal unit establishment; in another hospital, a nurse officially on the rota for neonatal unit work was actually undertaking a neonatal course at another hospital.

In addition to attending delivery suite, neonatal nurses are increasingly expected to work outside the neonatal unit. They may be asked to accompany babies to theatre and assist with recovery, be involved in transport to other units and run out-patient follow-up clinics or parent groups. In taking on these kind of activities, experienced staff are not available for direct care and they can be away from the unit for extended periods:

> 'At night squad calls cause real problems. We work with 6 staff, 4 trained & 2 nursery nurses. With a squad call a very experienced nurse must go, leaving only 3 trained staff with up to 27 babies, some very unstable and perhaps 6 ventilated. The childrens intensive care ward has one nurse per child/baby.'

> 'The pressure of work changes rapidly and although you can commence a shift with adequate staff, by the end the situation can be quite different.'

At hospital or unit level responses to nurse staffing problems are often short term, reacting to crisis situations and sudden fluctuations in workload. Reviews of nurse staffing and activity analyses (using workload audit systems) must include these and other factors in the estimates arrived at, if they are to be more than a purely paper exercise and bear a real relationship with the 24 hour care needed for small, sick babies.

The phenomenon of relatively small district units carrying out intensive care on other than a purely short-term basis, referred to in the House of Commons Health Committee Report (1992) was recorded during this study. This makes the medical and nurse staffing of these units more critical and the need for accreditation or specific criteria and practice guidelines more urgent (CSAG, 1993; BAPM, 1995). The implications of running unfunded intensive care cots are serious and may have immediate and longterm consequences for the staff trying to manage and for the babies and their families. The admission of older children and babies to neonatal units when local paediatric care facilities are absent or inadequate also has an impact on the organisation, staffing and the delivery of care in neonatal units. This includes practical consequences such as the added infection control measures required for treating non-neonates and effects on staff of trying to address the psycho-social needs of a different client group and their families.

Recent changes in hospital medical staffing associated with the need to reduce junior doctors' hours and workload and improve training have resulted in improvements in neonatal unit medical staffing and cover. However, the situation for nurses generally has changed little. Neonatal nurses in the many units studied clearly felt themselves to be under pressure, and from the data collected on staffing, this would seem to be an accurate perception of their present situation. Improvements in nurse staffing levels are needed generally so that all units begin to approach the more recently recommended levels (Redshaw, Harris and Ingram, 1993). Linked with this is the need for a more flexible mechanism for updating the establishment and calculating staffing requirements. To work, any formula must reasonably take account of the different types of leave, continuing education and training needs. Regular, at least annual, reviews of nurse staffing, linked to routine data-based workload information should be an integral part of the updating mechanism.

There is a pressure to link outcome with a number of factors including staffing and organization, however the nature of the intervening variables, the paucity of data available on the neonatal and post-neonatal periods and the lack of an agreed data set for follow-up, make this difficult (Mugford et al, 1988a, 1988b; Audit Commission, 1993). The need for rationalization of neonatal services has long been recognised (RCP, 1988; Dunn, 1988; BAPM, 1989; CSAG, 1993). Reasons for the present organisation and structure of neonatal care at regional, district and trust level are varied. Local conditions, historical precedents and powerful personalities have played their part and provision has not always been linked with local service need.

The Northern Neonatal Network report (1993b) has emphasised the benefits of inter-unit co-operation in dealing with workload fluctuations and of differently sized units working together, suggesting that with a flexible attitude and local agreement, fewer cots are needed. In the present study a large proportion of units were admitting babies for intensive care with no intensive care cots available (and the associated equipment and nursing staff). It seems that such co-operation and flexibility may not be practicable or possible everywhere, particularly in the present climate of competition, in which some small units fear for their continued existence. The push to obtain extra-contractual referrals or to avoid them, depending on what size of unit is being run, may influence the extent of cooperation. Geographically isolated units also present practical problems as far as co-operation is concerned.

The degree of understaffing or overstaffing depends on the model or standard adopted for the number of nurses or doctors required. The models examined may not be agreed, acceptable or appropriate, yet they provide a useful means of making inter-unit comparisons. Dependency and activity studies have been undertaken in some units in an attempt to produce alternative patient-linked means of setting nurse staffing levels (James et al, 1991; Northern Neonatal Network, 1993; Williams et al, 1993). Comparable data on medical staffing using similar methods are as yet unavailable, though with the pressure to reduce junior doctors hours, such studies will undoubtedly be forthcoming (Greenhalge, 1994). Accurate, up-to-date information is needed as the basis for decision-making and planning in neonatal care, as in other expensive, technical, labour-intensive areas of the health service. The staffing problems of acute specialties, where the peaks and troughs in patient numbers make planning difficult, require versatile mechanisms for budgeting and a fast response mode to deal with shortfalls in skills or numbers. To some extent more co-ordinated approaches to unit staffing problems within trusts are beginning to appear as a consequence of directorate groupings. In a few areas a more proactive strategy of cooperation, in some instances between trusts, is already at work: for example large units have joined and been functioning as one service and several smaller units have linked with a larger centre.

Alterations in unit status and an increasing desire to avoid transfer and to care for their inborn babies, especially those requiring intensive care, will necessitate a re-examination of the skill mix and team structure, especially with regard to teaching, maintaining and updating of skills. The idea of a critical mass or minimum throughput of babies requiring intensive care for individual units has been raised recently (British Association for Perinatal Medicine, 1995). In this rapidly changing specialty, the issue of training and education is an ever important one. The need for adequate numbers of experienced and qualified nurses in all types of unit, in all parts of the country, to care for sick newborns and their families has been widely acknowledged. Yet in practice there is a continuing disparity between this objective and what is found at the point of service delivery.

References

Arthur, T. and James, V. (1994) Determining nurse staffing levels: A critical review of the literature. *Journal of Advanced Nursing*, **19**, 558–566.

Audit Commission (1991) The Virtue of Patients: Making the Best Use of Ward Nursing Resources. HMSO, London.

Audit Commission (1993) Children First. HMSO, London.

Audit Commission (1995) The Doctors' Tale: Report on Medical Staffing. HMSO. London.

British Association for Perinatal Medicine Working Group (1989) Referrals for neonatal medical care in the United Kingdom over one year. *British Medical Journal*, **296**, 169–172.

British Paediatric Association (1993) The Care of Critically Ill Children. Report of the Working party on Paediatric Intensive Care. BPA. London.

British Association of Perinatal Medicine, RWIC/JLM, Report of Working Group of the British Association of Perinatal Medicine. (1992) Categories of Babies Requiring Neonatal Care. BAPM/BPA, London.

British Association for Perinatal Medicine (1995) Standards for Hospitals Providing Neonatal Intensive Care. Draft Report.

British Paediatric Association and British Association for Perinatal Medicine. (1984) Categories of Babies Receiving Neonatal Care. Circular DH/JG, BPA, London.

British Paediatric Association and the Royal College of Obstetricians and Gynaecologists Standing Joint Committee. (1983) Midwife and Nurse Staffing and Training for Special Care and Intensive Care of the Newborn. BPA/RCOG, London.

Clinical Standards Advisory Group, (1993) Access and Availability of Specialist Services. HMSO London.

Court Report. (1976) Fit for the Future. Report on the Committee on Child Health Services. HMSO. London.

Department of Health. (1989) Survey of Nurses in High Technology Care. NHS Executive. London.

Department of Health. (1993) Hospital Doctors: Training for the Future. Report of Working Group on Specialist Medical Training, Health Publications Unit, London.

Dunn, P. M. (1988) Medical and nurse staffing for the newborn. *Archives of Disease in Childhood*, **63**: 98–99.

English National Board for Nursing Midwifery and Health Visiting.(1987) Guidelines to the staffing of Neonatal Units. ENB, London.

English National Board for Nursing, Midwifery and Health Visiting.(1991) Guidelines for Staffing of Neonatal Units. Circular 91/09/APS, ENB, London.

Gray, A. M. and Phillips, V. L. (1994) Turnover, age and length of services: A comparison of nurses and other staff in the National Health Service. *Journal of Advanced Nursing*, **19**, 819–827.

Gray-Toft, P. and Anderson, J. G. (1981) Stress among hospital nursing staff: its causes and effects. *Social Science Medicine*, **15a**: 639–647.

Greenhalge and Company. (1994) The interface between junior doctors and nurses: A research study for the Department of Health.

Hawley, C. A. and Stilwell, J. A. (1993) The myth of the mid-day shift overlap. *Journal of Nursing Management*, **1**, 57–67.

Higginson, I. (1992) Description and preliminary evaluation of the Department of Health initiatives to reduce junior doctors hours. NHSME Report, London.

Hingley, P. and Cooper, C. L. (1986) Stress and the Nurse Manager. Wiley, Chichester.

House of Commons Health Committee (1992) Report on Maternity Services, Volume I, HMSO, London.

Jones, J., Black, N. and Sanderson, C. (1993) Levels of nurse staffing. *Senior Nurse*, **13**, 1, 20–24.

Jones, J., Sanderson, C. and Black, N. (1993) Does labour substitution occur in district general hospitals ? *Health Trends*, **25**, 68–72.

Mugford, M, Szczepura, A., Lodwick, A. and Stilwell, J. (1988) Factors affecting the outcome of maternity care I Relationship between staffing and perinatal deaths at the hospital of birth? *Journal of Epidemiology and Community Health*, **42**, 157–169.

Mugford, M, Szczepura, A., Lodwick, A. and Stilwell, J. (1988) Factors affecting the outcome of maternity care II Neonatal outcomes and resources beyond the hospital of birth. *Journal of Epidemiology and Community Health*, **42**, 170–176.

Northern Neonatal Network. (1993a) Measuring neonatal nursing workload. *Archives of Disease in Childhood*, **68**, 539–543.

Northern Neonatal Network. (1993b) Requirements for Neonatal Cots. *Archives of Disease in Childhood*, **68**, 544–549.

Redshaw. M., Harris A., and Ingram. J. (1993a) Nursing and medical staffing in neonatal units. *Journal of Nursing Management* **1**, 221–228.

Redshaw. M., Harris A., and Ingram. J. (1993b) The Neonatal Unit as a Working Environment: A Survey of Neonatal Unit Nursing. Executive Summary DOH London.

The Royal College of Physicians. (1988) Medical Care of The Newborn in England and Wales. RCP, London.

Sheldon Report. (1971) Report of the Expert Group on Special Care Babies. DHSS Reports on Public Health and Medical Subjects, 27, HMSO, London.

Walker, C. H. M. (1983) Special and intensive care baby units and nurse staffing in the UK. *Archives of Disease in Childhood*, **58**, 387–392.

Williams, S., Whelan, A., Weindling, A. M., and Cooke, R. I. W. (1993) Nursing staff requirements for neonatal intensive care. *Archives of Disease in Childhood*, **68**, 534–538.

Chapter 4 · Nursing Skill Mix

Mixing and Matching

The quality of nursing staff caring for small sick babies and their families is as important as the numbers of nurses employed in neonatal care. Concerns about staffing in neonatal units rest on a number of issues including overall numbers of nursing and medical staff employed. Adequacy and appropriateness of skill mix is also an issue in this acute specialty and in many other areas of nursing (Walker, 1983; Redshaw, Harris and Ingram, 1993; Redshaw and Harris, 1994). In order to run an acute service such as neonatal care effectively, a mixture of staff with varying experience, background and training are needed (DOH, 1989; Stock and Ball, 1993). The exact mix depends on many factors, including the type and number of babies cared for, the availability of nurses at a specific level, and financial constraints. It also changes over time as staff move, admission and staffing policies are changed and units are redesigned or combined.

The aim, in this area of the research was thus to investigate the structure of the workforce employed in the neonatal service as a whole and with reference to different types of neonatal unit, the shifts worked, particular responsibilities and duties undertaken.

Individual and unit data were thus collected on skill mix with the aim of examining the range and variety of different staffing structures and roles that were in operation. Nurses were also given the opportunity to express their views in their own words:

> 'The unpredictability of the workload results in staffing problems and there is a lack of understanding of this on the part of the nursing management at times of crisis. Poor skill-mix and inexperienced bank staff make up numbers, but create extra stress and frightening worries.'

> 'I only work two nights a week, and not always on SCBU. However, when I do, I am nearly always in charge of the unit and feel inadequately experienced for this.'

> 'The workload varies enormously from one shift to the next. Staffing is adequate for some shifts, but sickness and admissions can stretch the staff beyond acceptable limits.'

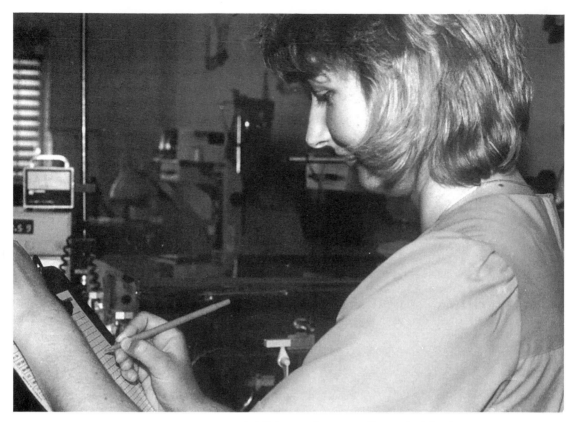

A skilled neonatal nurse recording routine 2-hourly observations in neonatal intensive care

In the first stage of the study the numbers of staff employed by title and grade in the 56 selected units were collected in order to investigate the range and variety of different staffing structures that were in use. At that stage details were returned on a total of 1890 nurses by grade and 1869 by title. In the second stage individual data were returned from 718 nurses working in twenty-four units. As reported in the methodology section (Chapter 2), little difference was found in the proportion of nurses responding individually in Phase II and the whole population examined in Phase I, either by unit type or by grade. Where results are presented below, reference will be made to indicate which data have been used in the calculations.

Skill Mix by Title

The distribution of nursing staff by title, across all the units surveyed is shown in Figure 4.1. From this, as might have been expected, it can be seen that staff nurses and staff midwives represent the largest segment of the workforce

(45%), followed by sisters (25%). The remainder is made up of nursery nurses (12%), enrolled nurses (10%), nursing auxiliaries (6%) and unit managers (2%)

The way in which the different types of unit employ nursing staff is shown by title in Figure 4.2. From this it appears that the relative proportions of the different types of staff employed differ little according to unit type. This was particularly true for the regional and sub-regional units. However, for the district units there was a slightly lower proportion of nurses in the staff nurse/staff midwife category (42% compared with 46%) and slightly greater numbers of enrolled (9% to 12%) and nursery nurses (10% to 16%).

In order to give a picture of the numbers of staff that may be employed in the different types of unit, Figure 4.3. shows the mean number per unit of the different categories of staff used by title. During the first stage of the study data were not collected on some aspects of staffing and a more detailed picture is provided by the Phase II information from individual nurses. The relative contributions of staff midwives and staff-nurses to the skill mix in neonatal care is shown in Figure 4.4. from which it is evident that overall, fewer staff midwives are employed in neonatal care than staff nurses. Examination of the data by unit type shows that district units were responsible for employing a significantly greater proportion of midwives than the larger units (p=<0.01). Some of these midwives are used as a flexible part of the workforce and a rotation onto the special care baby unit is part of their contract, while working on the labour or post-natal wards. However, some clearly have concerns and reservations about this:

> 'We have very few trained neonatal nurses. The midwives, myself included, are forced to rotate onto SCBU. We are neither properly trained or vocationally motivated, and as midwives, we feel that neonatal nursing is its own specialty, and is not a midwifery role specifically.'

> 'As a midwife I rotate onto SCBU without choice. I do not consider myself as a neonatal nurse and do not feel I have adequate training to cope when faced with many of the tasks allocated to me.'

The numbers of staff working as clinical teachers and clinical nurse specialists are also shown in Figure 4.4. That many of the regional and subregional units run post-basic neonatal courses accounts for the presence of nurses also being employed as teachers.

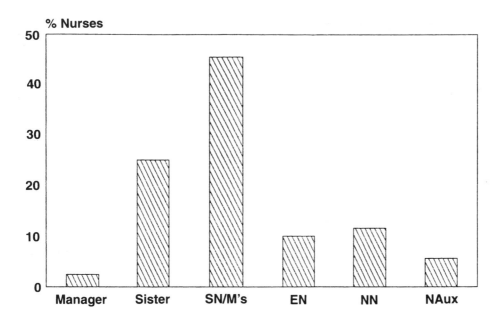

Figure 4.1 · Distribution of nursing staff by job title for all units combined (n=56 units, 1869 nurses)

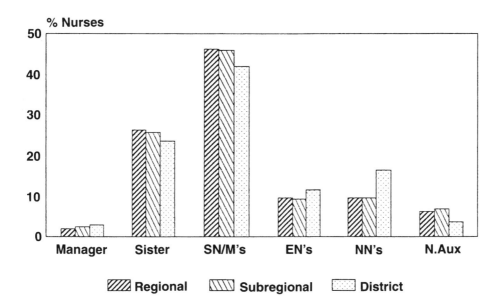

Figure 4.2 · Distribution of nursing staff employed by title in the different types of unit (n=56 units, 1869 nurses)

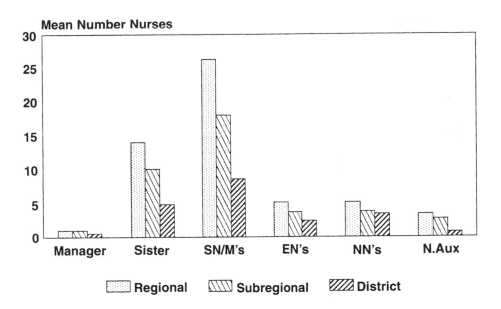

Figure 4.3 · Mean numbers of nursing staff employed by title in different types of unit (n=56 units, 1869 nurses)

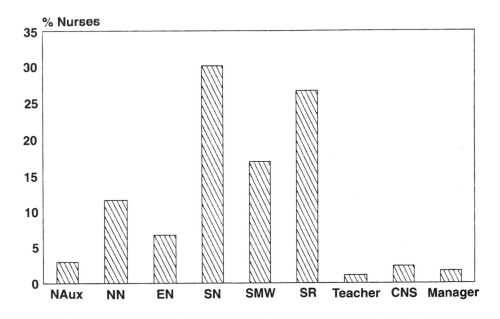

Figure 4.4 · Distribution of nursing staff by title including additional categories (n=24 units, 718 nurses)

Skill Mix by Grade

The breakdown of grades across all 56 units is shown in Figure 4.5. From the distribution of nursing staff by grade it can be seen that the E grade at 31%, the G grade at 19% and the F grade at 16% are the most frequently used. These are followed by the D at 12%, C at 9%, A and B both at 5% and H and I grades each at less than 2%. Figure 4.6 shows that the relative distribution of nursing staff by grade differed little between the regional and subregional units, though the latter employed more A grades. In contrast the district units employed more B grades, fewer E grades, slightly more F grades and as many G grades as the other types of unit. The mean numbers of staff at the different grades in the different types of unit are shown in Figure 4.7.

The question of just how closely the skill mix, as reflected by grade, matches the mix arising from title is an interesting one. Differences between the proportions resulting from classification of staff by title and by grade seem to indicate that different staffing policies may be in operation. The extent to which grades and titles match up is variable. For example, grade E was used for 31% of neonatal unit nurses, while staff nurses and staff-midwives represented 45% of the workforce. Similarly 19% of the workforce was employed at G grade, while 25% of the nurses working in the units were sisters.

Staffing Strategies

In order to address the question of policy or differential staffing strategies more directly, the data from each unit were examined to see which grades were and were not employed. Figure 4.8 a–c. shows the units one by one, grouped by type and ordered by the number of designated intensive care and then special care cots. It shows for any specific unit whether one or more nurses was employed at a particular grade.

Diverse staffing strategies were evident when these data from individual units were examined. Ten of the fourteen regional units in the study (Figure 4.8a) employed one or more nurses at both the H and I grades, while four units employed either I or H grades, but not both. Among the sub-regional units (Figure 4.8b.) there were fewer instances of employing both I and H grades. Ten units had one or the other and were as equally likely to have an I as an H. No district units (Figure 4.8c.) had both these grades, and indeed half of them had no unit staff at these levels at all. Where they were employed, the presence of I grade staff in a district neonatal unit was not associated with the size of unit or the type of care available there. With regard to the lower end of the scale there are less clear-cut variations. More than a third of units of all three types had no B grade staff. With few exceptions the regional and sub-regional units employed A grades, though nearly half of the district units did not employ this grade at all.

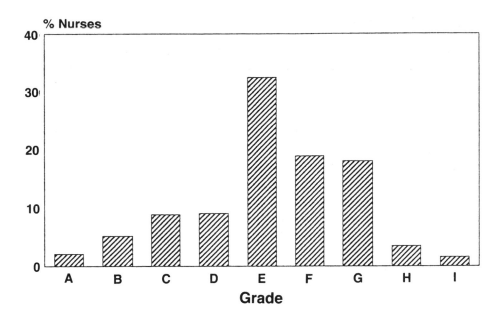

Figure 4.5 · Distribution of nursing staff by clinical grade for all units combined (n=56 units, 1890 nurses)

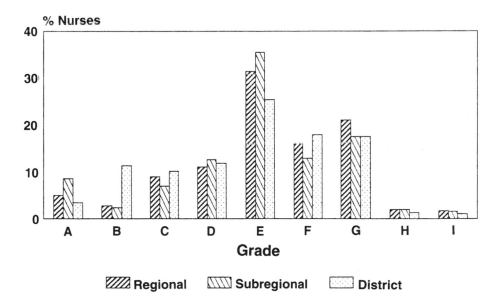

Figure 4.6 · Distribution of nursing staff by clinical grade for different types of unit (n=56 units, 1890 nurses)

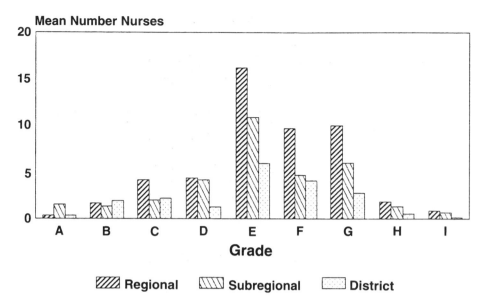

Figure 4.7 · Mean number of nursing staff employed at different grades in each type of unit (n=56 units, 1890 nurses)

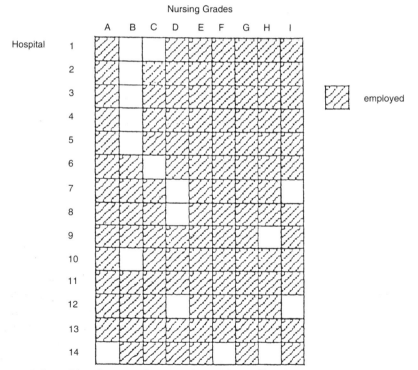

Figure 4.8a · Nursing grades employed in 14 Regional Neonatal Units (ranked in descending order by number of designated Intensive Care cots)

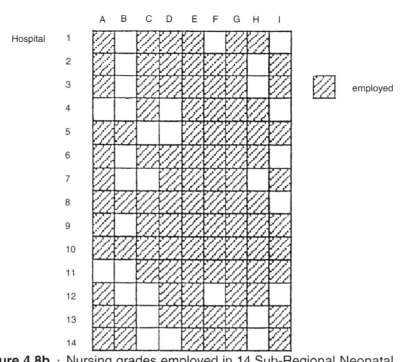

Nursing Grades

Figure 4.8b · Nursing grades employed in 14 Sub-Regional Neonatal
Units (ranked in descending order by number of
designated Intensive Care cots)

Inspection of the data by region showed some consistency for some grades, but in general there was little agreement. In grouping the data in this way few patterns and little consistency were observed. To illustrate the wide variation examples are given in Figure 4.9. for four different regions.

Where Are the Vacancies?

A total of 8% of nursing posts were reported to be vacant in neonatal care. The staffing levels at which these posts occurred are shown in Figure 4.10. From this it is evident that more than two-thirds of these were at the staff nurse and staff midwife level. The high technology survey (DOH, 1989) also found vacancies highest at this level. As staff nurses and staff midwives represent the largest proportion of the workforce, it is not surprising that vacancies should be found at this grade, but these were disproportionately high (p=<0.001). In terms of geography, the vacancies were quite widely distributed, with some bias towards the south-east, the Midlands and North West and as was discussed in Chapter 3, the majority of the vacancies were found to be in regional units both in 1990 and more recently.

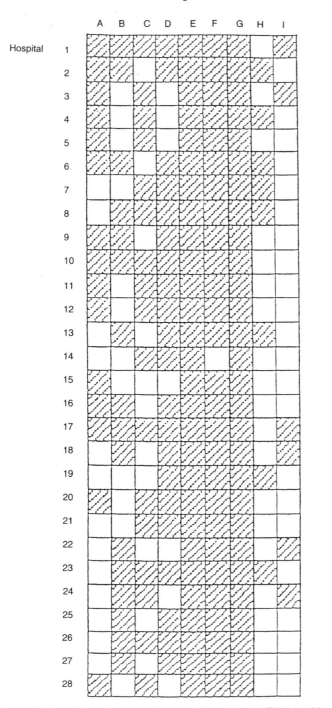

Nursing Grades

Hospital

Figure 4.8c · Nursing grades employed in 28 District Neonatal Units
(ranked in descending order by number of designated
Intensive Care and Special Care cots)

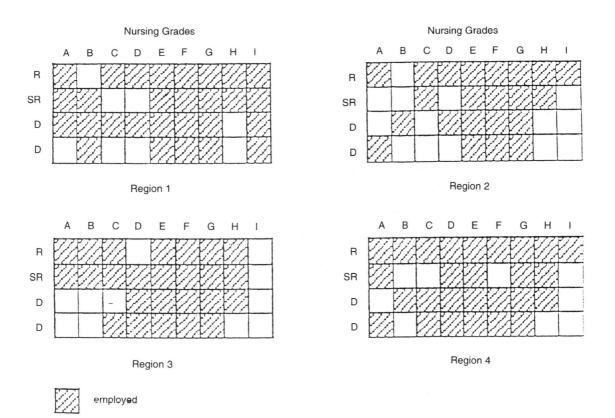

Figure 4.9 · Four examples of regional patterns of employment of nursing grades.
(R=Regional   SR=Sub-Regional   D=District)

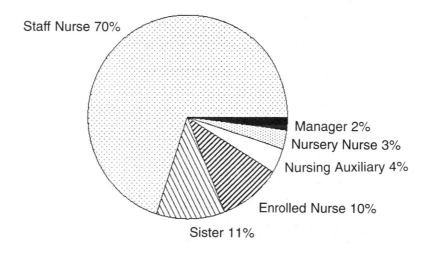

Figure 4.10 · Current neonatal nursing vacancies by title as a
proportion of the set establishment (% WTEs, n=56
units)

Skill-Mix and Shift

In Phase I details were obtained about the numbers of staff on duty on the early, late and night shifts. The way in which staff are deployed on these shifts in the different types of unit is shown in Figure 4.11 using the mean numbers of staff in the different categories from sisters to nursing auxiliaries.

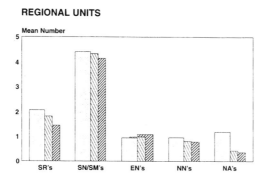

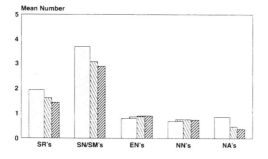

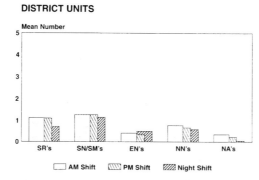

Figure 4.11 · Nurse staffing for the different shifts in the different types of neonatal unit (n=56 units)

There seems to be a common aim of maintaining a similar skill mix on the different shifts. However, the greatest numbers of staff are employed in the morning, followed by the afternoon and then the night shift. On average, in all three types of unit there is a reduction in the number of sisters and staff nurses and midwives as the day goes on and a small increase in the number of enrolled nurses employed. The tendency to employ more junior nursing staff at night is an important point to be considered in managing the skill mix in an area like neonatal care, where patient needs vary little with the time of day. Overall the skill mix of unit staff may be appropriate, but the wide variations in the mix available for some shifts and the concerns expressed by individual nurses indicate that there are very real difficulties to be overcome. The needs of sick babies vary little over the 24 hours and in planning the basic nursing skill-mix required for the different shifts it could be argued that the same mixture of skilled and experienced staff are needed for all three shifts.

Data from individual nurses indicated that 47% rotated, working both days and nights, but a significant proportion worked on days (25%) or on nights (28%). There was relatively little difference according to type of unit, with rotating staff predominating in large and small units. The distribution of these different staff by grade, however, varied significantly (Figure 4.12). Rotating between days and nights was highest for the middle grades; night shift work was highest for the lower end of the scale, though 16% of G grades were employed permanently on this shift; staff beyond this level generally worked day shifts, with a smaller proportion rotating.

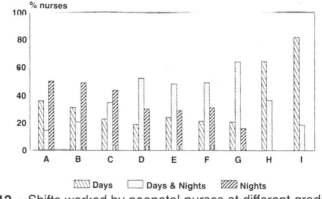

Figure 4.12 · Shifts worked by neonatal nurses at different grades (n=24 units, 718 nurses)

Roles and Responsibilities

Skill mix as characterised by grade is one way of differentiating the nursing staff, but a linear scale is necessarily a simplistic way of viewing the varying contributions to the skill mix needed in a neonatal unit. For many individual nurses their duties are complex and overlapping and they function in different capacities, at different times.

'100% of the time you are trying to do at least several jobs at once.'

'Senior nurses never "roll up their sleeves" and help out, no matter how short-staffed the unit is. We are expected to cope with whatever comes our way, including some of the jobs they should be doing'

'The staff nurses and sisters are highly competitive and the unit manager takes over on shift, rather than doing the managers' job'

In Phase II individual nurses were asked about their roles and responsibilities. Of the 718 nurses, 95% were currently working with babies, 20.5% were involved in unit management and 28% in teaching. The proportion caring for babies or involved in management varied little according to unit type, though fewer nursing staff were concerned with teaching in district units (23%, compared with 31% in the larger units).

As Figure 4.13. shows, nursing care was the main responsibility of nurses employed at A, B, C, D, E, and F grades. Involvement in this area was less than 100% of the higher grades, with 95% of G, 68% of H and 36% of I grades directly concerned with nursing care. Teaching responsibilities largely started with D grades, 10% of whom have some duties in this area, increased up to H grade and then declined. Management duties were not exclusive to the higher grades, though these were highest among the G and I grades.

Individual nurses were also asked about the job that they did, and whether it overlapped with the work of other hospital staff. Jobs for which most staff were over-qualified, and where their skills would seem to be inappropriately used, were as follows: 89% said they acted as ward clerk, 73% as domestics, 79% as nursing auxiliaries, and 55% as porters. Where other or more complex skills might be needed, a substantial proportion of nurses said they frequently took these on: the role of a secretary 83%, manager 82%, doctor 62%, and teacher

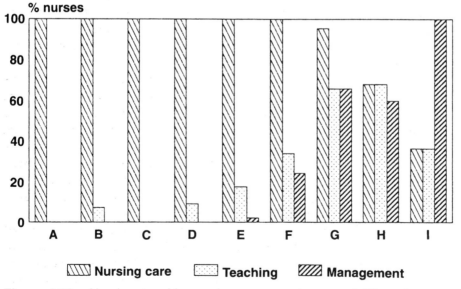

Figure 4.13 · Nursing, teaching and management responsibilities of nurses employed at different grades (n=718)

58%. This is an alternative account of "skill mix", in which neonatal nurses are multi-skilled individuals, "acting up" or down, or even laterally, as the situation requires. Skilled nurses are carrying out some duties that require little in the way of their specialised training and experience, but the need for them to do so depends on a number of factors, historical, organisational and personal. Examples are discussed in a section below on the nursing tasks actually undertaken by staff at different levels.

Unit Staff Other Than Qualified Nurses

It is clear that the skill mix required amongst the nurses working on a neonatal unit to some extent depends upon the support staff that are available to carry out some of the duties otherwise assigned to nursing staff.

Ward clerk duties may include answering the telephone, dealing with samples, handling records and entering data onto the record system, all of which in their absence usually fall to nurses to carry out. However, though valued for their contribution in this area, ward clerks are not routinely employed in neonatal units. All the regional centres, and almost all the subregional centres in the study, had at least one ward clerk, but most of these were employed on only a part-time basis and were often shared with other departments. Nearly half the district units had no ward clerk assistance at all.

Medical technicians were found to be employed in only eleven units, including both regional and subregional centres, and three units had more than one. The majority (45 units) had none. These staff have direct responsibility for equipment, or else are responsible via a Medical Physics Department and their duties can include setting up and calibrating equipment, equipment maintenance, some servicing and repair and staff training. As reports on the roles of nurses and technicians in high technology clinical areas (Youngman et al,1988; Stock and Ball, 1992) have indicated, there is considerable overlap in these areas between the work of technicians and nurses.

A liaison health visitor was attached to 45 of the units and those without this important service (20%) were equally likely to be regional or subregional centres as district units. The role of supporting parents and families, near the time of discharge and at other critical moments, is one with which neonatal nurses are familiar. When under pressure or understaffed, this kind of assistance is much needed and valued. The same can be said of the role of the social worker, particularly those who are either unit-based or shared. In fact, only 30 of the study units (54%) had a social worker (11 out of 13 regional centres, 8 out of 14 regional centres and 11 of the 28 district units).

Nursing auxiliaries were employed in 39 (70%) of the study units, and in half of these they carried out "hands on" nursing duties. Otherwise, they were involved in activities such as stocking up, laundry and cleaning incubators: duties that in some units are carried out by nurses. In fact, of the total of 1869 nurses identified by title as working in the fifty-six study units, 325 (17%) were not qualified and were working as nursing auxiliaries or nursery nurses.

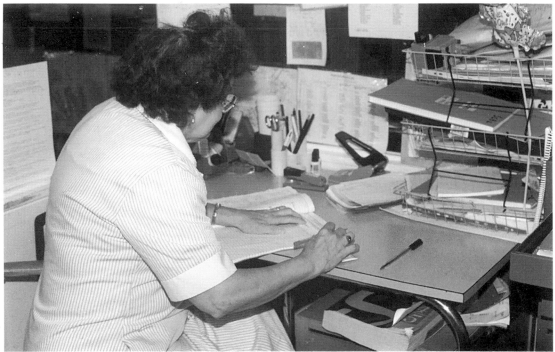

Support worker carrying out clerical duties in neonatal care

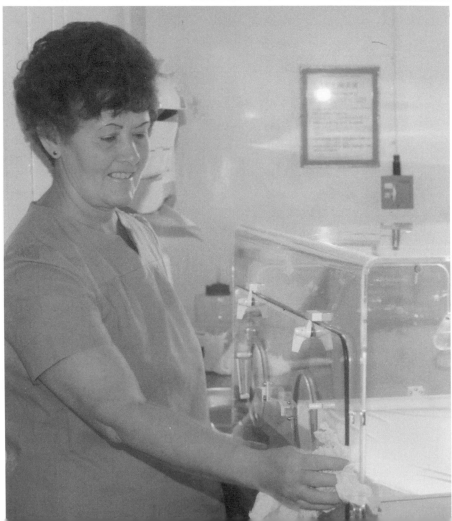

Housekeeping duties carried out by a nursing auxiliary

The study was carried out at a time of change in the role of the nursery nurse. Although there seems to be, in some units, an explicit policy whereby nursery nurse posts are not filled and nursery nurses are redeployed, they were still present on more than 80% of the study units. Indeed one unit employed as many as sixteen nursery nurses, justifying doing so out of necessity. However, in some units nursery nurses felt exploited, undervalued and "put on the scrap heap":

'I feel very frustrated because I am not allowed to do certain tasks that I was able to do in the past.'

'I am a nursery nurse of 20 years standing on a SCBU. I am saddened to see our role eroded and eliminated. Whilst accepting the situation as regards newly qualified nursery nurses, I do feel it is a waste of resources to discard experienced and loyal employees.'

'I have had to learn to accept the role of cheap labour. I would like my skills recognised as I am good at what I do.'

Nursery nurses have been, and in many units continue to be, a valuable part of the workforce in neonatal care. Their positive contribution was acknowledged by managers and fellow staff in the course of the study. However, as the role of non-nursing staff develops, the position of nursery nurses is changing and ultimately many senior nurses feel that in the neonatal unit of today there is little room for unqualified staff. The pressure, felt in some units currently, to employ health care assistants seems at variance with this view.

Learners on placement in units contribute by carrying out variable proportions of the work load, while at the same time as less experienced and unqualified individuals they can make demands on the resources of the permanent staff. By far the most frequent types of learner were student midwives and midwives on an update rotation, who had relatively little or no experience of the more specialised neonatal nursing tasks. Qualified nurses and midwives undertaking neonatal nursing courses were usually considered a valuable resource where courses were being run. This was the case for all but one of the regional units, half the sub-regional units and none of the districts units.

Nursing Tasks Undertaken

In order to understand more fully the nature of the role of the neonatal nurse, staff were asked to complete a task inventory. The topics covered ranged from basic care to dealing with parents and relatives, teaching, management and the more specialised nursing tasks. Subjects at all grades, and from different types of unit, responded to the same set of items and indicated the frequency or recency with which they undertook particular tasks. As a result a detailed picture of the work of nurses across the different grades and types of unit was obtained.

When the data were examined, there appeared to be little, other than quantity, to distinguish the work of the district units from that of regional or sub-regional units. However, when considering the work done by nurses in district units where there were no officially funded intensive care neonatal cots, it is apparent that the repertoire and range of tasks performed was little different from that of their counterparts in units with intensive care funding. Tasks carried out by nurses in district units without such funding included: caring for babies that were being ventilated, receiving paralysing agents, having an umbilical arterial catheter in situ, having a central venous pressure or long line, with a chest drain in situ, receiving peritoneal dialysis, with a tracheostomy and following major surgery. Many of these tasks would go beyond the requirement that such district units have of being able to provide short-term intensive care.

When looking at the areas of work covered by nurses at different grades, it became evident that there is much overlap in terms of who is carrying out which specific tasks and how often. Some neonatal nurses may be overqualified for some of the day-to-day activities examined eg. damp-dusting and cleaning incubators. However, in taking a task-oriented approach to the data collection, it is possible that the degree to which this occurs may have been exaggerated. Some tasks, like those mentioned, may be undertaken in a wider context such as preparing for a new admission. While some duties such as bottle feeding may be undertaken by senior staff to "help out" during a particularly busy shift, others such as checking the stores or the linen cupboard may be undertaken when a short period of "time out" is needed.

The important question of whether some unqualified staff were carrying out inappropriate tasks was also examined. (Harris and Redshaw, 1994). From the data collected, and in the course of visits to the individual units, it was clear that unqualified junior nurses were involved in caring for very small and sick babies. Among the tasks carried out by the staff working as nursing auxiliaries at A grade was caring for babies having additional or low flow oxygen, those with transcutaneous or saturation monitoring, babies with arterial monitoring lines in situ, weighing less than 1000 g. and following major surgery. Some A grades were also taking heel-prick blood-samples for serum bilirubin or blood sugar estimation (see Chapter 6). In comparing the range of tasks performed by nursing auxiliaries with nursery nurses employed at B grade, it was found that the latter group were undertaking the same tasks and some additional items. These included caring for babies undergoing ventilation, exchange or top-up transfusions, and those needing close observation.

Update on Skill-Mix

The skill mix in operation for neonatal care in 1994 in the main appears to be little different from that found during the study. Some nurses have been down-graded as part of a skill-mix review and others have chosen to be employed at a lower grade for "quality of life" or other personal reasons. Some units have been described as "grade rich" by senior hospital management and thus there has been a move to dilute or water down the mixture of staff employed. In some units of all types, as senior nursing staff have moved on or retired early, the opportunity has been taken to employ either only an H or I grade nurse rather than both grades of staff. In a number of units senior posts now also cover areas other than neonatal care, thus managers may be jointly responsible in the areas of maternity or paediatric care.

There has also been a change for some unit managers, whose responsibilities now lie in management, rather than clinical work. At the same time more F grade nurses are regularly expected to be "in charge", run the shift and allocate the care of babies, including their own. At the opposite end of the scale changes have also occurred, with smaller numbers of nursery nurses and nursing auxiliaries being employed in directly caring for babies. Plans for the introduction of health care assistants to the neonatal service, as mentioned above, have been discussed by senior management, but none were as yet employed in the 24 units for which data were collected in 1994.

Concurrently other roles are being considered such as that of "housekeeper" and parent support workers. At the other end of the spectrum in terms of technical and clinical skills is the advent of a new role, that of the advanced neonatal nurse practitioner (Hall et al, 1992; Redshaw and Harris, 1995) which seems to mark a new development in terms of the nursing skills available in neonatal care. However, the present availability and distribution of advanced neonatal nurse practitioners is limited, as relatively few cohorts have so far completed the course and qualified as practitioners in this specialty. (The changing and expanding role of the neonatal nurse is described and discussed in some detail in Chapter 6.)

Skill Mix, Skill Muddle ?

As in other research studies (Jones et al, 1992) variations in neonatal care were found between hospitals in the skill-mix in operation as characterised by title and by grade. Though there were differences, on the whole the mix of staff used appeared to be most similar in the two larger types of unit. In many ways subregional units seemed to be smaller scale versions of regional centres. This is perhaps not surprising in that their roles and the type of babies cared for are likely to be similar. However, district units seem to be run differently in this respect, with slightly more staff at lower grades and fewer support staff. Changes can be expected in this area, if in the future, smaller district units are going to carry out intensive care on other than a short-term basis.

Deciding on the appropriate overall skill-mix for an individual unit is a difficult task. It depends on many factors including the goals and professional standards adopted, the variations in workload that occur, the staff available and the budget to pay for them. Maintaining an appropriate skill mix on a day-to-day basis, taking into account the needs of the current babies and others that might be admitted, is a yet more complex task involving as it must leave, off-duty and other requirements. The benefits of employing other forms of staff to work in neonatal units, in addition to those with medical and nursing qualifications should perhaps be considered seriously by those not yet using them. An integrated multidisciplinary team, with a wide range of clinical and other skills is more likely to be able to pursue and reach the goals embodied in the written philosophies of care that are increasingly being put forward.

Changes in unit status and an increasing desire to avoid transfer and to care for their inborn babies, even those requiring intensive care for less than 24 hours, will necessitate a re-examination of the present skill mix and team structure in many units, particularly with regard to teaching and updating skills. The use of unqualified staff to carry out tasks preferably allocated to qualified and trained nurses has practical, legal and other service implications in both the short and long term. Clinical practice supervision of the quality required for unqualified and non-specialty trained nurses by senior experienced staff (Butterworth and Faugier, 1992) is in many instances impractical in the context of current unit lay-out and design. The use of such staff, "supervised" or not, while carrying out the kind of tasks mentioned is of considerable concern (Harris, 1995). Skill mix requirements need to be taken into account if accreditation mechanisms and guidelines are to be set up and implemented (Audit Commission, 1993; BAPM, 1994).

In addition to differing service demands that may affect the skill mix required, there is a clear need for the profession to address the questions that arise from substitution, changing roles and areas of responsibility in the spheres of management, teaching, supervision and clinical practice (DOH, 1994).

In conclusion, there is much talk of skill mix, but in many instances, the debates are about grades rather than skills and about costs rather than the quality of care provided. The wide variation between units, even those of a similar type and size indicates that a realistic examination is needed of the kind of skill mix required in neonatal care. This is particularly evident in relation to more technically oriented expanded role skills and those involved in basic infant care. A re-evaluation of the role of unqualified nursing staff is required in relation to the nursing of babies requiring intensive and high dependency care. At the same time it is important to recognise the valuable role that nursery nurses and auxiliaries have played in the past and to plan realistically for the future, especially in the light of the pressure to employ health care assistants in acute areas like neonatal care.

It seems that what is included within the scope of neonatal nursing is a wide range of duties and responsibilities, only some of which are reflected in the grades at which individuals are employed. Neonatal nurses appear to be multi-skilled, taking on a wide range of nursing and other jobs. Some appear to be carrying out tasks that require little of their specialised training and experience, though the therapeutic benefits of carrying out duties such as tidying the linen cupboard should not be underestimated. At the same time some nurses are taking on work and areas of activity that have been considered to be the preserve of junior medical staff (Chiswick and Roberton, 1987; Hall et al, 1992; Harris and Redshaw, 1994). This is another aspect of what is meant by "skill mix" in the area of neonatal care and like the role of unqualified nursing staff will also need to be addressed more fully if skill mix is to mean more than just the crude numbers of nurses that can be employed at the different grades.

References

Audit Commission (1993) Children First. HMSO, London.

British Association for Perinatal Medicine (1994) Standards for Hospitals Providing Neonatal Intensive Care. Report in Preparation.

Butterworth, C. A. and Faugier, J. (1992) Eds. Clinical Supervision and Mentorship in Nursing, Chapman and Hall, London.

Chiswick M. and Roberton C. (1987). Doctors and nurses in neonatal intensive care: towards integration. *Arch. Dis. Childhood*, **62**, 760–763.

Department of Health. (1989). Survey of Nurses in High Technology Care. NHS Management Executive.

Department of Health (1994) The Challenges for Nursing and Midwifery in the 21st Century. DOH, London.

Hall, M., Smith, S., Jackson, J., Perks, E. and Walton, P. (1992) Neonatal nurse practitioners – a view from perfidious Albion?. *Archives of Disease in Childhood*, **67**: 458–462.

Harris, A. (1995) The Expanding Role of the Nurse in Neonatal Care. Unpublished MSc thesis. University of Bristol.

Harris., A. and Redshaw (1994) The changing role of the nurse in neonatal care: A study of current practice in England. *Journal of Advanced Nursing*, **20**, 874–880.

Jones, J., Black, N. and Sanderson, C. (1992) Levels of nurse staffing. *Senior Nurse*, **13**, 1, 20–24.

Northern Neonatal Network. (1993a) Measuring neonatal nursing workload. *Archives of Disease in Childhood*, **68**, 539–543.

Redshaw, M., Harris, A., and Ingram, J. (1993) Nursing and medical staffing in neonatal units. *Journal of Nursing Management* **1**, 221–228.

Redshaw, M. and Harris, A. (1995) An exploratory study into the role of the advanced neonatal nurse and the educational programme of preparation. Report to the English National Board for Nursing, Midwifery and Health Visiting.

Stock, J. and Ball, J. (1993) A Study of Nurses and Technicians in High Technology Areas. IMS Report 240, Brighton.

Walker, C. H. M. (1983) Special and intensive care baby units and nurse staffing in the UK. *Archives of Disease in Childhood*, **58**, 387–392.

Youngman, M., Mockett, S. and Baxter, C. (1988). The Roles of Nurses and Technicians in High Technology Areas, Preliminary Report, DHSS, London.

Walker, C. H. M. (1983) Special and intensive care baby units and nurse staffing in the UK. *Archives of Disease in Childhood*, **58**: 387–392.

Chapter 5 · Training and Education

Education for Care

The issue of nurse education and training is a paramount concern in the context of providing a high quality service for small, sick babies and their families. In this relatively recent and fast developing specialty, the issue of training and education is an increasingly important one. The skills required for neonatal nursing today are diverse: technical equipment must be set up, used and maintained; complex fine motor tasks must be carried out while caring for small dependent patients and social skills are needed to provide and promote effective support and communication with both parents and colleagues.

The need for experienced and qualified nurses caring for sick newborns has been widely acknowledged (BPA, 1983; DOH, 1989; ENB 1987; RCP, 1988; BAPM, 1992; Audit Commission, 1993). Yet in practice it is evident that there are contradictions between what is considered optimal and the current situation; the theoretical levels of qualified staff and the skill mix actually available overall and on each shift. Nurses themselves are only too aware of the deficiencies in this area:

> 'It is worrying that qualified and experienced neonatal nurses have left the unit, only to be replaced by unqualified and inexperienced staff nurses'

> 'An 11th intensive care baby was admitted into ten spaces when we were short of staff and already using a nursery nurse in intensive care as she was the most experienced of the mix of agency and nursery nurses that we had at the time. The less experienced nurses were left to look after high dependency babies'

> 'I am a new member of staff on the unit and I often feel I am placed in situations that I am too inexperienced to handle'

For part of this study of neonatal nursing data were collected from both unit managers and individual nurses. The managers and senior nurses from all 56 units (100%) returned general information on staffing numbers, training and facilities. Individual nurse data collection entailed a specific section on training and education that covered a wide range of topics including educational background, age at entry to neonatal nursing, professional qualifications, experience, orientation, appraisal and update. The same nurses were also able to make additional comments if they wished.

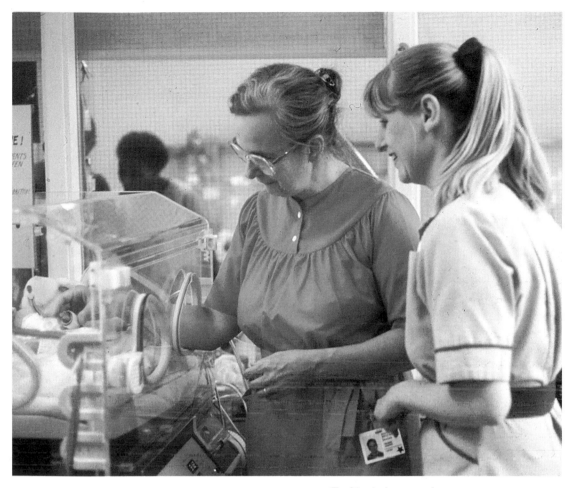

Teaching in the neonatal area

Educational Background

The level of general education reached by the 718 nurses working in this specialty was relatively low: the majority of neonatal nursing staff (58%) reached O-level or GCSE level; a smaller number had taken A-levels and very few (3%) had taken a degree. Age at entry to neonatal nursing is shown in Figure 5.1. The majority of staff began work in neonatal care between the ages of 20 and 30 years (69%), but a substantial number entered the specialty at a later age (20% between 30 and 40, and 7% after the age of 40 years).

Trained and Qualified Nurses

Any nursing team responsible for the care of babies in a neonatal unit has members that are qualified and practised and others with less training and experience. Data collected on the numbers of trained and qualified nursing staff working in the 56 study units indicated that of the 1869 identified by title 17% were not trained and registered nurses and were working as nursery nurses or nursing auxiliaries (Redshaw and Harris, 1994). The extent to which untrained staff were employed in the different types of neonatal unit varied little, with regional centres having 84% staff qualified, subregional units 83% and district units 80%.

Nursing Qualifications

Individual nurses were asked about their nursing qualifications and a full list of these is shown for each type of unit (Table 5.1). Three-quarters of individual nurses had qualified as registered nurses (RN) and 45% as registered midwives (RM). Fewer staff (17%) were registered sick children's nurses (RSCN), enrolled nurses (9%) (EN) or nursery nurses (15%) (NNEB). Many nurses had more than one basic qualification (Table 5.2), though the degree of overlap was variable. For example, of the RMs 97% were also RNs and 8% RSCNs, but of the RNs a smaller proportion (58%) were midwives and a slightly greater proportion (20%) were registered children's nurses.

Nurses with a Qualification in Specialty

Nurses who held the English National Board neonatal courses (ENB 405, 409, 904 and earlier versions of these) were categorised as being qualified in specialty (QIS). Of the 1869 nurses employed in the 56 units, only 44% had undertaken these courses and were thus qualified in specialty. However, if only trained nurses are included, ie. not nursery nurses or nursing auxiliaries, the proportion of nurses that were QIS rises to 53%. A significant difference was found between the different types of unit (p=<0.001) (Figure 5.2), the proportions of QIS nurses in regional, subregional and in district units being 50%, 49%, and 32% respectively.

QIS rates for different levels of staff were examined: for all types of unit the level of QIS for managers and sisters was similar at 80% and 82%. However, the rate for staff nurses and staff midwives was half that (41%,) and even lower for enrolled nurses (28%). In comparing the rates for the same level of staff in the different types of unit (Figure 5.3) relatively few differences were found: a

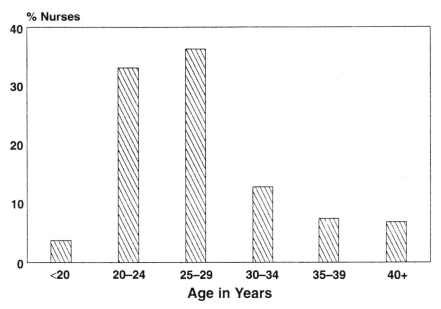

Figure 5.1 · Age on entry to neonatal nursing (n=718 nurses)

Table 5.1 · The proportion (%) of nursing staff with different qualifications in the different types of unit

Qualification	UNIT TYPE			
	Regional (n=294)	Subregional (n=195)	District (n-229)	All units (n=718)
None	1.7	4.6	3.0	2.9
NNEB	12.2	11.8	19.7	14.5
EN	10.9	6.7	8.7	9.1
RN	78.9	75.9	71.5	75.7
RSCN	21.4	19.5	11.4	17.7
RM	45.2	36.9	51.3	44.9
Diploma in Nursing	2.7	1.5	0.9	1.8
Diploma in Midwifery	0.3	0.5	0.5	0.4
JBCNS 400*	4.8	3.1	0.4	2.9
JBCNS 401	1.0	1.0	0.9	1.0
JBCNS 402	5.1	3.6	7.5	5.4
ENB 405	34.7	25.6	15.8	26.2
ENB 409	1.4	1.0	–	0.8
ENB 904	2.7	5.6	4.8	4.2
ENB 998	7.5	3.6	4.4	5.4
ENB 997	7.1	6.2	8.3	7.3
RCNT†	0.7	–	–	0.3

* JBCNS Joint Board of Clinical Nursing Studies
† RCNT Registered Clinical Nurse Teacher

Table 5.2 · Details of neonatal nursing staff with more than one basic qualification showing the extent (%) of overlap

Qualification	NNEB	EN	RN	RM	RSCN
NNEB n=104		6.73	14.42	5.77	1.92
EN n=65	10.77		27.69	24.62	1.54
RN n=543	2.76	3.31		57.64	19.89
RM n=322	1.86	4.97	97.20		7.76
RSCN n=127	1.57	0.79	85.04	19.69	

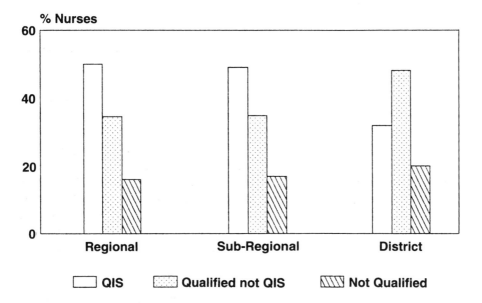

Figure 5.3 · Nursing staff qualified in the specialty (QIS) in the different types of unit (n=56 units, 1869 nurses)

slightly lower proportion of managers in regional and district units were QIS than in subregional units and relatively fewer QIS staff nurses, midwives and enrolled nurses employed in district units. Overall the pattern was similar with lower grades of staff being less likely to have a qualification in specialty. Nevertheless, the rates found did indicate an increase since 1981, when only 36% of sisters and 15% of staff nurses working in this specialty were reported to have had additional formal training (Walker, 1983).

Large inter-unit differences were found in the proportions of nursing staff qualified in specialty in the 56 initial study sites. The rates across all three types of unit ranged from 0–79% of staff: in regional centres the QIS rate was between 26–73%, in subregional centres 17–79% and 0–68% in district units (Redshaw, Harris and Ingram, 1993). The lower level of QIS staff in district units was reflected in the lower proportion of nurses undertaking neonatal and other courses at the time (7% compared with 11% for the larger centres).

The rates of QIS found in this study are higher than those reported in a survey of nurses in high technology care (DOH, 1989). The difference may be a function of slightly increased numbers of nurses with a post-registration qualification, but also due to the different samples of units used (see Chapter 2). In comparison with the 1989 DOH survey, fewer of the very smallest district units were included in the present study.

Who is Qualified in Specialty?

Data on QIS and clinical nursing grades are shown in Figure 5.4. A clear relationship with seniority was found, with G and H grades having the highest QIS rates, followed by F and I grades. QIS rates were also examined in relation to age. These were found to be significantly different for the various age groups (p=<0.001): the rate was highest among the 30–39 year olds (50%), followed by nurses aged 20–29 (26%), 40–49 (19%) and those aged 50 years and over (6%).

The lower level of QIS in district units is reflected in the lower proportion of nurses undertaking neonatal and other courses. From these data it would seem to be some time before these units could reach the 70% QIS rate put forward by the English National Board for Nursing, Midwifery and Health Visiting (1991). However, some progress has been shown by the study on high technology care (1989) which recorded 61% of sisters, 13% of staff nurses and staff midwives and 21% of enrolled nurses working in neonatal units as qualified in specialty.

In this same population the relationships between having a qualification in this specialty and the type of work nurses were contracted to do (full-time or part-time, and days, nights or rotating days and nights) were examined. Significant differences were found in QIS rates on both aspects (p=<0.001). For those working part-time the QIS rate was half that of nurses working full-time (25% compared with 52%) and of all the nursing staff qualified in

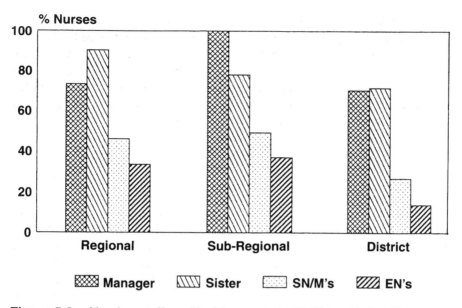

Figure 5.3 · Nursing staff qualified in specialty (QIS) by title in different types of unit (n=56 units, 1869 nurses)

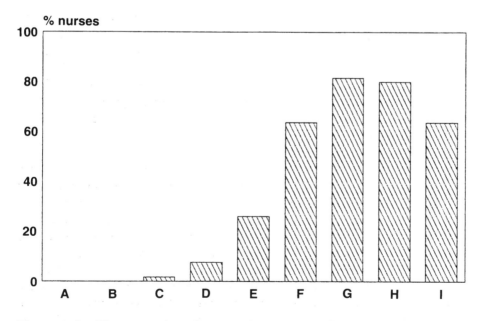

Figure 5.4 · The proportion of neonatal nurses at different grades that are qualified in specialty (n=718 nurses)

specialty 30% were part-time workers. In terms of shifts, nurses rotating between days and nights had the highest QIS rate (52%), followed by those on days (35%) and then those on nights (25%). The low rate of QIS among the night staff fits in with other study data concerning differences between the staff employed on the different shifts (Chapter 4). It appears that the high rate for staff rotating between shifts indicates that they are to some extent being used as a means of improving the mix and counteracting the night shift difference.

Update on QIS

More recent data collection on qualification in specialty generally indicates little change in this area. Additional information collected from 24 units in 1994 shows that in comparison with the overall rate of 53% found in the main study the rate of 52% does not represent an improvement since 1990. The previously marked difference between the different types of unit was less evident than before. However, large inter-unit differences were still present: the regional units for which data were collected ranged from 30–53% QIS, subregional from 44–74% and district units from 24–77%.

The Role of Experience

The age structure of the population of neonatal nurses generally seems to resemble that reported for nurses as a whole (Seccombe and Ball, 1992), with the majority being between twenty and forty years of age. It seems probable that with their relatively high levels of post-basic training the population of neonatal nurses may be slightly older on average, however, since different response categories were used, direct comparisons are not possible. When the data are examined by unit type (Figure 5.5) it is noticeable that slightly greater proportions of younger nurses are employed in the regional units, followed by the subregional and then the district units.

Of the nurses working in neonatal care who do not have a qualification in this specialty, many have years of practical experience in caring for small, sick babies. In the second stage of the study, data were collected on the total duration of time that individual nurses had been employed in neonatal care.

The nursing staff studied had worked in neonatal nursing for periods ranging from one month to thirty-five years, with a mean of 7.4 years and a median of 5.1. years. The distribution of time spent in neonatal nursing for all subjects is shown in Figure 5.6. Most of the staff (57%) had five or more years experience in this specialty, though 9% had less than a year. Differences between regional, subregional and district units in this respect are illustrated in Figure 5.7. Years of experience in relation to grade are illustrated in Figure 5.8. The details shown reflect a mixture of factors including the grades at which individuals commonly enter this specialty, the points up to which some progress or at

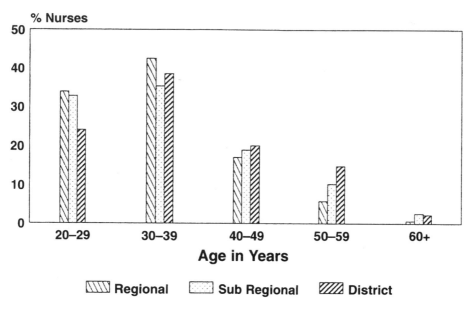

Figure 5.5 · The age of neonatal nurses working in different types of unit (n=24 units, 718 nurses)

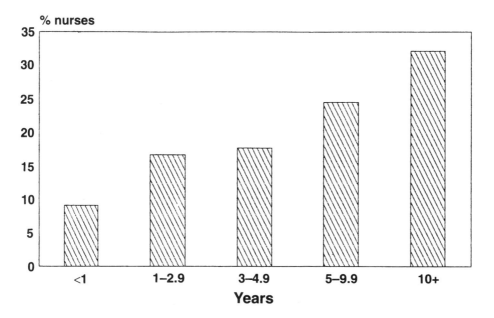

Figure 5.6 · The proportion of nurses working in neonatal care with different amounts of experience (n=718 nurses)

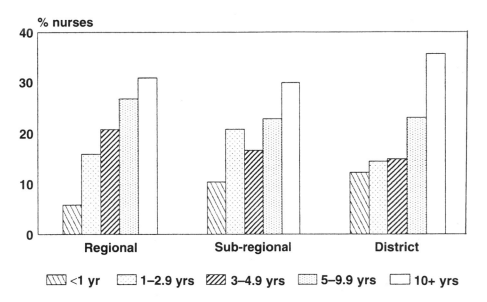

% nurses

⬜ <1 yr   ▧ 1–2.9 yrs   ▨ 3–4.9 yrs   ▦ 5–9.9 yrs   ⬜ 10+ yrs

Figure 5.7 · Years of neonatal nursing experience of nurses working in different types of unit (n=718 nurses)

which others may stay. The more neonatally experienced staff dominate at the higher and lower ends of the scale, at one end being nursery nurses or auxiliaries of longstanding and at the other being neonatal nurses experienced and trained in the specialty who have progressed up the clinical ladder.

The time spent by any nurse in the present unit in which she or he is working is likely to reflect both experience and mobility more directly than the total time spent working in neonatal care. Amongst the individual nurses the mean time spent in their present unit was 5.9 years (median 4 years), with a range of one month to twenty-six years. The distribution is a fairly even one across the categories shown in Figure 5.9, but with slightly more nurses in the longer duration categories. Figure 5.10. shows the distribution of these over the different types of unit, with all three types presenting a similarly even picture, except for relatively greater numbers of staff staying longer in the smaller district units. An examination of duration of stay according to grade (Figure 5.11) shows that across all units grades A, B, and C and G, H. and I have stayed for the longest times. As might be expected D, E, and F grades were the more mobile grades, perhaps being those with more family and other commitments, as well as the group most likely to go on courses.

The benefits of cross-fertilization that come with the introduction of new staff can be great, especially where changes are needed and senior medical staff have been in post for many years. In order to gain an impression of the breadth of experience of nurses working in neonatal care, individual nurses were asked about the number of units that they had worked in, including training units. Of the population of nurses studied 73% had only worked in one or two units (68% for regional centres, 79% for subregional units and 74% for district

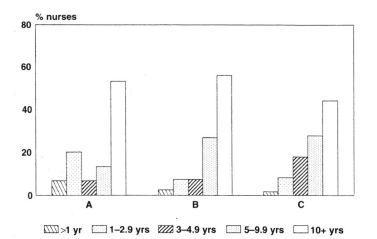

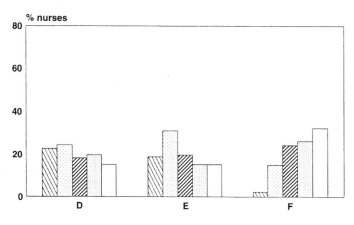

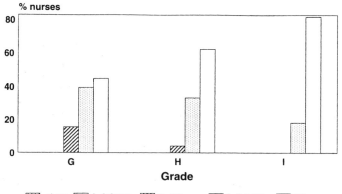

Figure 5.8 · Years of neonatal nursing experience of nurses at different clinical grades (n=718 nurses)

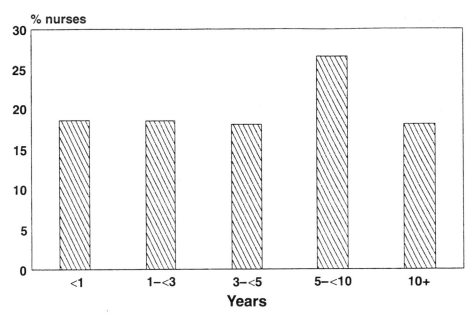

Figure 5.9 · Years worked by nurses in their present unit (n=718 nurses)

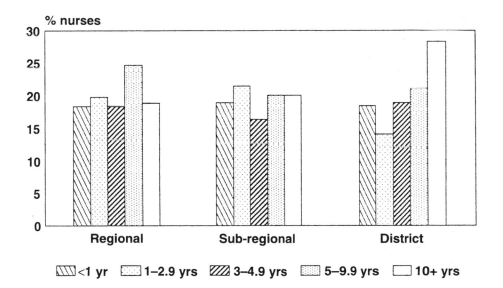

Figure 5.10 · Years worked in present unit by nurses employed in different types of unit (n=24 units, 718 nurses)

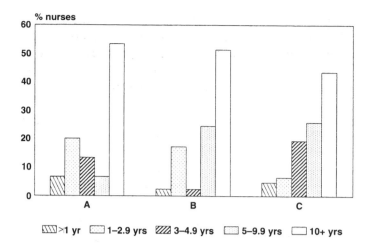

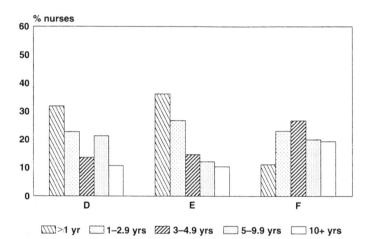

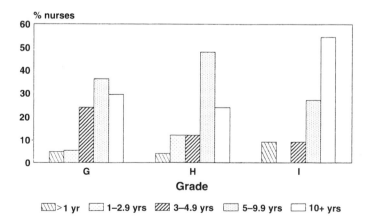

Figure 5.11 · Years worked in present unit by nurses at different grades (n=718 nurses)

units). However, amongst the 27% that had worked in more units, there were a small number who had worked in as many as seven units, some of these abroad. Mobility seems to increase with grade up to a point (Figure 5.12) for no A grades and only 10% of Bs had worked in three or more different units, compared with 40% of G grade and more than half of the nurses working at H grade.

A total of 9% of those surveyed had gained experience working outside the United Kingdom, though of course these are nurses that have returned to work in England after being abroad. The majority (39%) went to the Middle East, 25% to Australia and smaller numbers to other parts of Europe, the United States of America, Canada and the Far East. The nurses with this kind of experience were not evenly distributed across the different types of unit; they were 13% of nurses working in regional centres, 7% of those in subregional units and 6% of neonatal nurses in district units. This could mean that staff are returning to what might be considered a more technologically oriented work situation or just a function of greater employment opportunities in the largest units where vacancies are higher.

From the data on the numbers of units worked in, the years spent in the present unit and in neonatal nursing, it would seem that the nursing workforce is more stable than might have been expected based on reports of turnover and retention (DOH, 1989; Gray and Phillips, 1994). However, the group of nurses that participated in the study may contain a higher proportion of those committed to the profession. A survey of nurses who have taken the different neonatal courses with follow-up at spaced intervals afterwards, as well as the collection of exit data by hospitals, might provide information on the costs of training and the long-term retention of qualified staff in the profession.

Undoubtedly there is a segment of the neonatal nursing workforce that work in one or two units for the major portion of their working lives. Whether this is done out of a sense of loyalty and commitment, convenience and expediency, or as a consequence of coming to neonatal nursing at a more settled stage in life is uncertain. The effect is that, in conjunction with staffing policy changes, many of which apparently have an underlying financial rationale, many nurses feel that promotion prospects and experience are limited in their present unit:

'This particular unit is stagnating. There are no opportunities for promotion, and because of the high number of sisters, no chance of gaining management experience.'

'I have just joined the unit as an E grade. I feel there will never be any chance of promotion here, due to the numbers of senior staff here already.'

'Many staff here are unhappy about the lack of promotion prospects, it is difficult to motivate and support them.'

'The manager and senior sisters here all stick together in "the crows' nest". There is little or no chance of promotion while they are in control.'

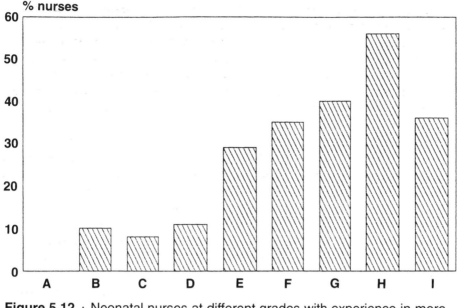

% nurses

Figure 5.12 · Neonatal nurses at different grades with experience in more than two units (n=718 nurses)

Among the individual nurses 375 were able to give reasons for leaving their last post. Career and job related reasons were high among these: a job change in order to secure promotion (18%); a move for training and secondment (15%); following training (7%); better conditions of work (9%) and a change of career direction (7%). If retention of experienced and trained staff is really seen as a problem, it would seem that strategies related to career development need to be worked out that take account of some of these factors.

Orientation and Up-date

Obtaining a qualification in the specialty is only one aspect of training. How an individual nurse is introduced to a unit, supported and subsequently up-dated are important aspects of continuing education in fast-changing, highly technical specialties.

Individual data on nurses joining their unit in the last five years showed that 65% had been given an orientation programme and this proportion differed little by unit type. Programmes ranged from less than a day to more than three months and the majority (55%) lasted less than a week. However, those in regional centres were generally longer, the median being three weeks, compared with one week for both subregional and district units. There was a significant difference in the provision of mentors for new staff (p=<0.001): these were most frequent in regional centres (64%), less so in subregional centres (39%), and least common in district units (25%).

Orientation was slightly more likely to have been provided in the larger centres (56% nurses working in regional centres, 54% subregional and 47%

district units). More than a third of the staff at each grade had received an orientation programme, though these were more often given to the D and E grades than others, 65% and 63% of whom had orientation programmes.

Some of the staff had clearly joined their units at a time when orientation programmes were not as current as now. In order to have an up-to-date picture of the recent situation, the data on those joining their unit in the last five years were examined separately. Of these, 65% had been given an orientation programme. This differed little by unit type, though there was a significant difference with regard to the provision of mentors. This was most frequent in regional centres which provided 64% of new staff with another member of staff in this role, less so in subregional units (39%), and least frequent in district units (25%). When the duration of programmes was examined, not surprisingly, those given in regional centres were significantly longer than the other types of unit. Considerable inter-unit variation was found, the median for regional units was three weeks and one week for subregional and district units. These frequencies, based on the experience of individual nurses, are lower than those reported by managers and senior nurses in Phase I. At that time, 91% said that an orientation programme was in operation, and a mentor system was said to be provided in 89% of units. Based on this information it seems that either a large proportion of nurses are missing out on orientation somehow, or that the Phase I responses of managers were overly optimistic.

The individual nurses were also asked about other things that helped them settle in. For the majority (81%) the answer lay in the support of other members of the nursing staff. Experience on the bank prior to employment, staff development programmes clinical teachers and study days were also mentioned. The last of these is an important way of nurses hearing about new developments in their profession, however, not everyone is given or takes the opportunity to go to these:

> 'It is difficult to get permission to go on a study day in our unit, and even more difficult to get funding for one.'

> 'If you work part-time, you don't stand much of a chance of going on courses or study days.'

In fact, only 54% of nursing staff had been on one or more study days in the previous two years, and there was little difference in the proportions attending according to unit type. However, with the advent of PREP (The Post-Registration Education and Practice Project, UKCC, 1990) the situation is likely to be changing, with increasing numbers of staff attending or being required to attend increasing numbers of study days.

Of the individual nurses surveyed in Phase II, 27% indicated that they were currently waiting to take a post-basic course. For most (33%) these were the longer neonatal nursing courses (the ENB 405 and 409); 15% were waiting to do the short three week neonatal course (ENB 904), while others (17% and 21% of those waiting) were hoping to do the more teaching oriented courses (ENB 997 and 998). Other courses included nursing degrees, RSCN and advanced nurse practitioner courses. The expected waiting time ranged from less than a month to more than a year, and nearly half (46%) expected to wait six months and more before beginning a course.

However, once on, or following a course, not everything is straightforward:

'As a 405 course student from another unit I have found that this one lacks basic standards and guidelines, let alone professionalism. I am rapidly losing zest and enthusiasm for the work here. I don't feel I can or should lower my standards to their levels.'

'Most of the staff on the unit have worked here for years. They dislike and feel threatened by change. The girls who do the 405 course leave because they are not allowed to use the new skills they have gained.'

Nurses not being able to exercise the skills for which they have been trained was a recurring theme throughout the study.

Appraisal and Professional Development

Staff appraisal is an important aspect of nursing management; the opportunity for positive feedback and review is considered an integral feature of staff management in many professions today (Ansty, 1971). Yet in many neonatal units, though the concept has been agreed in principle, there is no staff appraisal system in practice, or it operates selectively for some grades of staff only.

'I have only been working as a neonatal nurse for 3 months and am still feeling insecure and not terribly confident. You only get feedback when your performance is unsatisfactory. Thanks are important and make the difference between going home unappreciated and feeling valued.'

'I would like better assessment. Appraisal means PRAISE as well as being told when we have ERRED.'

A situation in which the relative strengths and weaknesses of individual nurses are discussed directly with them and in which they are also given the chance to say how they see their present position and career possibilities is a valuable forum for discussing future training and development. In the first part managers indicated that 63% of units had a system of appraisal interviews for staff. In the second, 61% of the individual nurses asked about an appraisal system on their unit, said there was such a scheme in operation. However, of these nurses less than half (47%) had been appraised in the last year, 18% between one and two years previously, 10% more than two years ago and though a system was officially operative, 26% were still waiting. Even less common was the use of professional development plans, for only 19% of nurses reported having such a plan as part of their appraisal and review system, though nursing management claimed that these were used in 64% of units. It may be that this difference can partly be accounted for by appraisal being used selectively for some grades, but this would not account for the magnitude of the discrepancy found.

In a profession that has a history of being hierarchically organised, with distinct professional roles and responsibilities and established mechanisms for dealing with errors and problems, one might have expected the more widespread adoption of appraisal. However, the apparent slowness to acquire and develop management, as well as specialty nursing skills, may account for this tardiness. A need for support, training and update for managers was also evident:

'I have previously worked in a big unit. I am now working as manager in a much smaller SCBU and finding the lack of resources hard to adjust to. My main concern is the reluctance of older members of staff to update their policies and care. This includes the consultants as well as the nursing staff.'

'The manager has recently been promoted and takes over on shift, rather than doing her own job.'

'The management are out of touch. They treat the staff like school children. At the same time we are expected to be totally dedicated to the job.'

'We would like more recognition for the hard work that is carried out looking after such small, sick babies. Hardly anyone in management says "thank you".'

'I love my job, but there are times when I wish the managers would pay more attention to what we, the nurses actually giving "hands on" care, have to say.'

The gap between managers and other nursing staff is one of which the neonatal nurses studied were clearly aware: feelings of alienation and frustration were evident. Problems with role definition are common and more senior staff frequently described feeling caught between demands of the hospital management and the needs of the other nursing staff working on the unit. In being promoted to a more senior position and in adopting some of the management role, loyalties may be switched, or divided:

'On the whole I enjoy the work, but find the constraints imposed by management sometimes very unrealistic and very frustrating. Everything is down to cost-cutting, imposing a greater workload and more paperwork or computer work, when we should be beside the babies in their incubators.'

Many managers in moving on from the senior sister's role are ill-prepared for what they have to take on; their clinical and nursing skills in many cases matter less than their ability to concern themselves with budgeting, fund-raising and managing change. Among those who feel most insecure are nurses who have achieved the position as a function of seniority and nursing experience, rather than any intrinsic interest in this changing area within the health service. Some may have been moved on when their clinical skills did not match up with what is required in clinical practice. A need for support, training and update was explicitly expressed by managers themselves. Promotion, often from within their own unit, resulted in difficulties in changing and defining roles and drawing new professional boundaries. The evolution of the multi-skilled nurse manager out of the senior sister's role has had a dual effect, creating the possibility of greater scope for professional development while adding other pressures.

The quality of communication between managers and other levels of nursing staff often seemed quite poor and was commonly unidirectional. Changes were presented as a "fait accompli" and partiality in selection for courses and promotion were common concerns. In the face of these problems many nurses did not feel heard, or listened to. From this kind of situation it is but a short step to the feelings of powerlessness and apathy encountered, that in turn can only affect the working environment adversely.

Quality and Quantity

Education and training in neonatal care, whether in-service or as a course, is dependent on the skills and abilities of the staff actually working in the units. There is an underlying assumption that because nurses are skilled at their job, they will be good at supervising and passing on their clinical and nursing skills. In fact, some teaching is needed for all those expected to have a teaching role and to be responsible for learners. The effectiveness of the learning environment and mentorship are directly dependent upon the quality of that environment and the mentors available at the time. An environment in which the staff are already stretched by a heavy workload and other responsibilities is not likely to be conducive to effective mentoring or to enhance learning outcomes. Other issues that relate to the adequacy of neonatal units as learning environments are the clinical standards and practices in operation and on which the quality of what is taught depends. All these factors enter into the equation that for some nurses means a positive learning experience and the development of new skills, but for others a lowered morale and in some cases thoughts about leaving this area of nursing all together.

In comparison with other specialties, a relatively high proportion of nursing staff in neonatal care had undertaken a post-basic neonatal nursing course (DOH, 1989). However, qualification in specialty rates were lower than those recommended (ENB, 1991) and most importantly there were very large differences between units in the numbers of nurses or midwives with a specialist qualification. Difficulties in retaining staff once qualified and the availability of courses and funding may have influenced this situation. However, that some units had been obliged to drop the neonatal course or the number of student places as a consequence of their staffing situation is significant.

More generally a greater variety of courses to suit nurses at different stages and at different ends of the spectrum could ameliorate the situation. Until recently the choice has largely lain between a clinically-oriented practical course of approximately 24 weeks or a three week theoretical one. The development of other types and forms of course including the Advanced Neonatal Nurse Practitioner programme (Southampton College of Nursing and Midwifery, 1991), the modularisation of ENB 405 neonatal courses, the design of specialist distance learning packages and the development of "core" curricula show that other routes are developing. Changes in the organisation of nurse education and the separation of the institutions responsible for courses from those providing the clinical experience and training have created at least temporary uncertainties about the location of courses, availability and differences in curricula.

Many of the nurses working in neonatal care without a qualification in the specialty could gain from an increasing diversity of courses. One group of nurses who could benefit are those who are older than average, usually with a great deal of experience, often in one unit, who may feel unsuited for a longer course which is more oriented towards nurses with less practical experience. A shorter programme devised with the needs of this kind of group in mind, mixing theory and practice, could be a way of updating their knowledge and skills, as well as swelling the numbers of appropriately qualified neonatal unit staff. Another group whose clinical update needs seem relatively neglected are the midwives who work in neonatal care as part of a rotation. Addressing their educational needs in this area could do much to reduce the anxiety and concern expressed by those who felt inappropriately qualified to be working in a neonatal unit, particularly with babies requiring intensive care. The introduction of the "lecturer practitioner" may assist in bridging the theory-practice gap for a range of learners and qualified nursing staff, though the role itself has yet to be fully established and recognised.

Targeting units with low QIS rates, distributing courses more evenly in geographical terms and the allocation of places and funding aimed at increasing the QIS rates for specific units is a strategy that could be used to improve the picture presented to those purchasing or planning to purchase neonatal services.

From the more general perspective of considering educational needs in this area there is undoubtedly a place for exchanges and "out-reach" schemes which can address a range of update and training needs. Links between units of the same type and size and between small and large units are needed at service level and in the spheres of specialist education and professional development. A more coordinated and cooperative approach would be to the benefit of both large and small units from a number of aspects, including the costly area of education. Inter-unit differences in organisation, policy and standards of care could be reduced, while one would expect in-service training, update and professional support to improve.

Clear policy-practice gaps were found to exist in the areas of appraisal, orientation and professional development. With PREP (UKCC, 1990) the situation will change and increasing numbers of staff be required to attend a prescribed minimum number of study days. Statutory requirements will place both financial and other demands on individuals and institutions. These practical issues will need to be addressed if the numbers and range of staff attending study days are to be increased.

Education and training in neonatal care, whether in-service or as a recognised course depends on continuous input and supervision from the nursing and medical staff caring for babies in neonatal units, as well as those providing a more theoretical input. The staff carrying out the day-to-day care have a formative influence, providing role models and examples of practice. A need to diminish the policy-practice gap is evident.

The role of nurse manager is changing (Hingley and Cooper, 1989) and there is debate about the inclusion of a clinical nursing element. A manager who is clinically competent and understands the intricacies of neonatal care can provide a valuable source of expertise. However, there may be conflict between clinical and organisational or managerial responsibilities. Further training and development for nurses in this position is vital to empower them to cope effectively with the demands and pressures of the health service today. The need for the development of leadership skills and peer group support are great in this, as in many areas.

This part of the present study shows that a more systematic and yet imaginative approach to the development of training and skills is required in the area of neonatal care that takes account of the need for research, innovation and standards. The education needs of this group of nurse is high; they work in a rapidly changing field and need to keep up to date. If qualified nurses are to carry meaningful portfolios, undertake undergraduate and postgraduate degrees or courses in advanced specialist practice, there has to be committed organisational support and interest in their professional and educational development.

References

Ansty, E. (1971) Staff Reporting and Development. George Allen and Unwin, London.

Audit Commission. (1993) Children First: Improving the Health Care of Sick Children. London.

British Paediatric Association and the Royal College of Obstetricians and Gynaecologists Standing Joint Committee. (1983) Midwife and Nurse Staffing and Training for Special Care and Intensive Care of the Newborn. BPA/RCOG, London.

British Association of Perinatal Medicine. (1992) RWIC/JLM, Report of Working Group of the British Association of Perinatal Medicine. Categories of Babies Requiring Neonatal Care. BAPM/BPA. London.

Department of Health. (1989) Survey of Nurses in High Technology Care. NHS Executive, London.

English National Board for Nursing Midwifery and Health Visiting. (1987) Guidelines to the staffing of Neonatal Units. ENB, London.

English National Board for Nursing, Midwifery and Health Visiting. (1991) Guidelines for Staffing of Neonatal Units. Circular 91/09/APS, ENB, London.

Gray, A. and Phillips, V. (1994) Turnover, age and length of service: a comparison of nurses and other staff in the National Health Service. *Journal of Advanced Nursing*, **19**, 819–827.

Hingley, P. and Cooper, C. (1989) Stress and the Nurse Manager, Wiley, Chichester.

Redshaw, M., Harris, A. and Ingram, J. (1993) Nursing and Medical Staffing in Neonatal Units. *Journal of Nursing Management* **1**, 221–228.

Redshaw, M. and Harris, A. (1994) Nursing Skill-Mix in Neonatal Care. *Journal of Nursing Management*, **2**, 15–23.

Seccombe, I. and Ball, J. (1992) Motivation, Moral and Mobility. IMS Report No 233. IMS Brighton.

Southampton College of Nursing and Midwifery (1991) Course Outline.

The Royal College of Physicians. (1988) Medical Care of The Newborn in England and Wales. RCP, London.

UKCC. (1990) Post Registration Education Practice Project. Position Statement. London.

Walker, C. H. M. (1983) Special and intensive care baby units and nurse staffing in the UK. *Archives of Disease in Childhood*, **58**: 387–392.

Chapter 6 · Changing Roles, Changing Places?

Specialist and Developing Practice

During its evolution the field of neonatology has seen rapid advances in terms of the knowledge and expertise needed to care for increasing numbers of small sick newborn babies (Harvey, et al, 1989; Roberton, 1993; Audit Commission, 1993). Associated with this developing understanding and advances in technology, nursing and medical techniques have been refined. Nurses working in this area have developed a skill base from which to deliver both technical and practical care and this is now embodied in the post basic courses providing specific training in special and intensive care of the newborn.

Development of the nurse's role in neonatal care has taken place in a number of countries, commonly in response to medical staffing crises (Boxall, 1987). In the United States advancement of the role has largely taken place in a technical direction, encompassing a wide range of practical clinical procedures previously undertaken by medical staff (Harper et al, 1982; Karp, 1993). In Canada, although the role is clinically focused and contains a technical element, relatively greater emphasis appears to have been placed on expanding the nursing role in areas that include administration, teaching, parental support and research (Herbert and Little, 1983; Beresford, 1991). Interest in the concept of the advanced neonatal nurse practitioner in the United Kingdom has been developing (Chiswick and Roberton, 1987; Hale et al, 1987). Findings from a National Association of Neonatal Nurses survey about neonatal nurse practitioners concluded that while it was important to look to the future, there were reservations about development of the role (Boxall, 1987; Hall et al, 1992). Fundamental issues such as staffing adequacy, remuneration, career structure and the goal of delivering holistic family care needed to be addressed in addition to immediate training needs.

Recent studies in the United Kingdom have focused on the role of the nurse in high technology areas (DOH, 1989; Stock and Ball, 1992), looking at qualifications in specialty and the overlap between tasks carried out by nurses and technicians. The possibility of overlap in other areas is also evident, with increasing interest and concern on the part of professional bodies and organisations in the potential of advanced practice and the development of nurse practitioner roles. The concern and interest essentially spring from two different perspectives: one focused on the changing scope of the nurse's professional practice (UKCC, 1992), the other oriented towards the possibility of nurse practitioners taking on clinical duties normally assigned to junior medical staff in training (DOH, 1993; Higginson, 1993; Greenhalge, 1994; Audit Commission, 1995). The nurse practitioner role has been taken on by nurses in the community (Stilwell et al, 1987; Drury et al, 1988; Touche Ross, 1994) and is now being introduced in a wide range of hospital specialties including cardiovascular surgery, urology, paediatrics and accident and emergency care (Read and George, 1994; Trent Regional Health Authority, 1995). In the area of neonatal nursing an advanced practitioner course has been running for several years in one English health region (Hall et al, 1991; Redshaw and Harris, 1995) and others are being set up.

As part of this national study of neonatal nursing the issue of the changing role of the neonatal nurse was addressed specifically in relation to the "extended" and "expanding" role of the nurses studied. The extent to which nurses in the neonatal unit assist medical staff with procedures was also investigated.

In the course of hearing from nurses during the unit visits and among the study respondents as a whole, a wide range of views were expressed. A number of nurses, like those in intensive care units (Last et al, 1992), felt that they were assisting with procedures that, with appropriate training, could be better undertaken by themselves. This kind of feeling and concerns expressed about inexperienced junior medical staff carrying out procedures on small sick babies are obviously motivating factors in nurses seeking opportunities and training in which to expand their practice and at the same time improve the quality of care.

'New doctor month is stressful. SHO's all change at once. Many are inexperienced in the specialty or simply find the change difficult; they are tired and overwhelmed and so I am too! I have real anxiety at times over their decisions (or lack of them). I sometimes feel very anxious and responsible as they demand advice and support from me as an experienced nurse.'

'I was very concerned over the junior doctors' attitude to work, the medical management of certain babies and failure to come promptly when called to see a critically ill baby.'

The problems of availability and delays in procedures or administration of fluids or medication are among those specifically identified by nurses.

The Changing Role

In order to answer the question of how far the "extended" or "expanded" role is already in operation in the specialty, data were collected in the course of interviews with unit managers and individual nurses were questioned using a list of 30 tasks (Harris, 1995). These included methods of blood sampling, administration of drugs and a wide range of technical and invasive procedures. The nurses were asked whether they had undertaken the task in the past and whether they were doing so regularly now. If they had not yet carried out the task they were asked whether they wished to do so. This area of the task inventory was in addition to wider data collection on more traditional aspects of neonatal care nursing.

The data presented here on practice developments, unless otherwise stated, are those obtained on the 718 staff participating in the study of whom 599 were qualified nurses in the D–I grades. The effects of grade, unit type and qualification in specialty on the performance of specific tasks were examined. Data were also collected concerning 15 different medical procedures for which nursing assistance is commonly required. The extent to which nursing staff had recently been involved in these was examined separately for the different grades.

Policy on Expanding the Role

Interviews with nurse managers indicated that for only a quarter of units (6 out of 24) was there a policy regarding the expanded role. The units with such a policy included district as well as regional centres and were located in a number of health regions.

When asked about specific activities heelprick blood sampling by nurses was reported for all units, administration of intravenous (IV) antibiotics for 88% (21 units) and removal of intravenous cannulae for 83% (20 units). Intravenous administration of other drugs at 67% (16 units), intubation at 42% (10 units), use of a blood gas analyser at 63% (15 units) and use of a bilirubinometer at 42% (10 units) were less common. No unit managers reported nursing staff undertaking insertion of intra-arterial (IA) cannulae, umbilical arterial catheters (UAC) or chest drains.

Tasks Commonly Undertaken by Individual Nurses

The data collected on individual nurses show that tasks routinely carried out by those working in neonatal care and graded D–I include taking heelprick blood samples (90%), removing IV cannulae (89%), and giving IV antibiotics (67%). Higher proportions of nurses had actually carried out these tasks at some time, though were not doing so regularly: 98% heelprick sampling, 98% removing IV cannulae, and 77% giving IV antibiotics. The distribution for some tasks carried out by nurses graded D–I is shown in Figure 6.1. demonstrating a significant grade effect for the giving of IV antibiotics ($p=<0.001$), but little difference on the other tasks shown. When these data are displayed according to unit type (Figure 6.2.) few differences are evident.

Less Common Activities

Other less common tasks and areas of care in which some nurses in neonatal units were involved were also examined. Intravenous administration of drugs other than antibiotics was regularly undertaken by 50% of D–I grade nurses, removal of endotracheal (ET) tubes (as an emergency or elective procedure) by 44%, setting up of arterial blood pressure monitoring by 41% and removal of

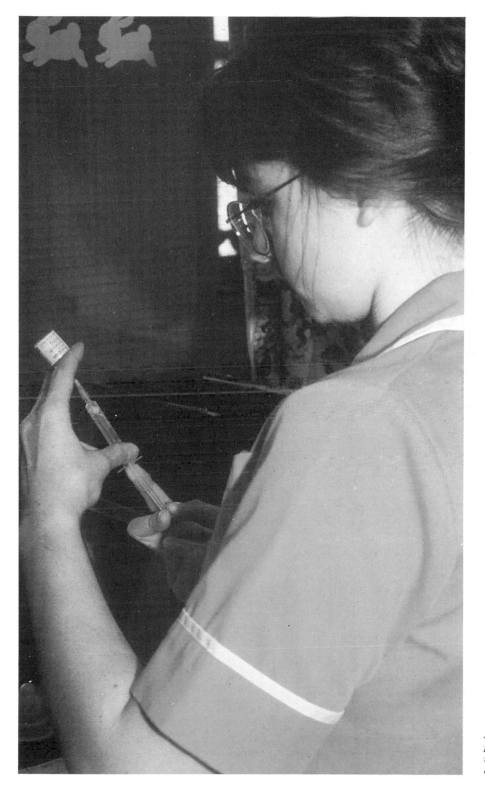

A neonatal nurse preparing drugs for intravenous administration

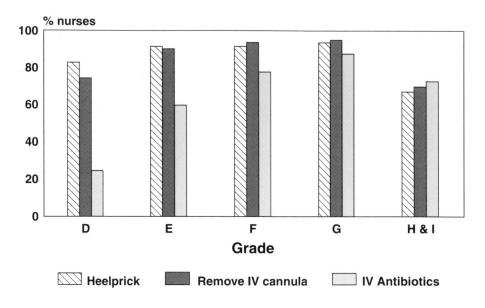

Figure 6.1 · Common tasks regularly carried out by neonatal nurses at grades D–I (n=599 nurses)

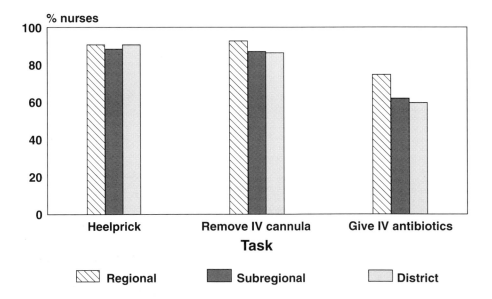

Figure 6.2 · Common tasks regularly carried out by D–I grade nurses in different types of unit (n=599 nurses)

peripheral IA cannulae by 38%. As with the more common tasks, greater numbers of nurses had carried these out previously, though were not doing so regularly now. At some time 65% of nurses had given drugs other than antibiotics intravenously, 80% had removed ET tubes, 66% set up arterial BP monitoring, and 66% removed peripheral IA cannulae.

Differences across the clinical grades in carrying out these tasks are shown in Figure 6.3. where there is a clear effect of seniority, with significantly more G grade nurses regularly undertaking these tasks than nurses at any of the other levels (p=<0.01–<0.001). Differences according to unit type are shown in Figure 6.4. The proportion of nurses carrying out these tasks was greatest in the regional centres, followed by the subregional and then the district units (p=<0.001), reflecting both the levels of care available and the type of babies admitted.

Other still less common tasks that were regularly carried out by 20% or fewer of D–I grade nurses were removal of an umbilical arterial catheter (20%), using a blood gas analyser (13%), using a bilirubinometer (12%) and taking a blood sample from an indwelling arterial catheter (9%). A frequency distribution by grade is shown in Figure 6.5. Similar significant effects of grade to those reported for more common tasks were found (p=<0.01) for all except use of a bilirubinometer. Some less obvious effects of unit type were found, for example, the use of a bilirubinometer was actually higher for nurses working in subregional and district units (21% and 19% compared with 2% in regional centres).

The tasks that were most infrequently reported as a routine part of the neonatal nurse's work are shown in Table 6.1. From these data it appears that a small proportion of nurses in neonatal care are carrying out a range of tasks that have more usually been carried out by medical staff. It is also evident that some nurses had in the past performed procedures that they are not currently undertaking.

Nurses Qualified in the Specialty

It was reassuring to find that in general nurses with a post-basic qualification in the speciality were carrying out the tasks examined more often than those without a post-basic qualification. However, for the two most common activities (heelprick sampling and removing IV cannulae) being QIS made little difference. Of all the staff carrying out heelpricks 48% were qualified in the specialty and the comparable figure for nurses removing IV cannulae was 51%. For all the other tasks examined, including the giving of antibiotics intravenously, there was a significant relationship with having a post-basic neonatal qualification (p=<0.001 for all but use of the blood gas analyser and the bilirubinometer, for which the significance levels were p=<0.01 and p=<0.02 respectively). The proportion of QIS nurses undertaking the less common tasks was quite high and varied relatively little between the tasks, ranging from 61% of nurses using a bilirubinometer to 75% of those taking a blood sample from an indwelling arterial catheter.

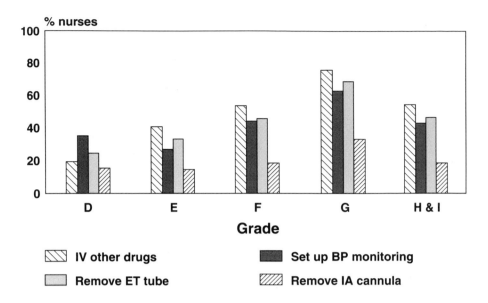

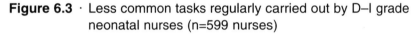

Figure 6.3 · Less common tasks regularly carried out by D–I grade neonatal nurses (n=599 nurses)

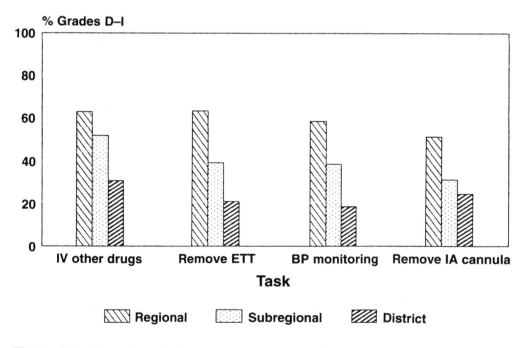

Figure 6.4 · Less common tasks carried out regularly by neonatal nurses in different types of unit (n=599 nurses)

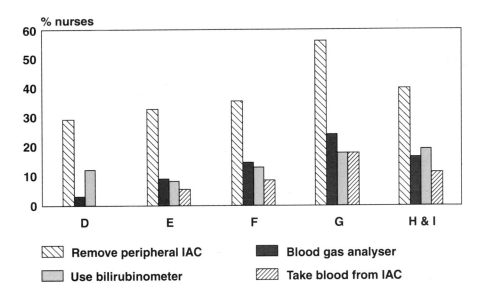

Figure 6.5 · Other less common tasks regularly carried out by D–I grade neonatal nurses (n=599 nurses)

Table 6.1 · Tasks carried out infrequently by neonatal nurses grades D–I (n=599)

TASKS	% Nurses carrying out task regularly	% Nurses having carried out task previously
Venepuncture	1.17	12.19
Arterial stab	0.33	1.50
Insertion of IV cannula	1.67	11.02
Insertion of IA cannula	0.33	0.67
Insertion of U.A.C.	0.17	0.50
Insertion of C.V.P. catheter	0.17	0.17
Intubation	1.67	21.54
Insertion of chest drain	0.50	1.00
Removal of chest drain	4.84	24.87
Lumbar puncture	0.17	0.17
Calculation of T.P.N. requirements	0.50	3.84

A–C Grade Junior Staff

Data were also collected from the A–C grade staff on the same range of tasks. Of the 119 staff in the study at these grades, most were nursery nurses or nursing auxiliaries and only eleven (employed at C grade) were enrolled nurses. Heelprick blood sampling had been carried out by more than 80% of the staff at these grades; 52% had removed an IV cannula and 15% had used a bilirubinometer. More rarely some staff at these grades had undertaken administration of IV antibiotics, removal of an ET tube, removal of an IA cannula and used a blood gas analyser. The use of A–C grade nurses to carry out these tasks was not found to occur more commonly in any particular type of unit.

Overall there appeared to be relatively little, other than quantity to distinguish the work of the district units from that of regional or sub-regional units. When considering the work done by nurses in district units it was apparent that the repertoire of tasks performed was little different from that of their counterparts in units with greater capacity and funding for neonatal care. From the data collected on the types of babies individual nurses had cared for, and while observing in the course of visiting the units, it was clear that junior nurses were involved in caring for very small and sick babies. Some nurses at junior level (A grade nursing auxiliaries) had recently cared for babies in a wide range of situations: some in additional or low flow oxygen; having transcutaneous or saturation monitoring; with arterial monitoring lines in situ; babies born weighing less than 1000 g. and following major surgery. They were also taking heel-prick blood-samples for serum bilirubin or blood sugar estimation. A comparison of the range of tasks performed by nurses employed at A grade with those at B grade (nursery nurses), showed that some of the latter group were undertaking the same duties and others in addition. These included caring for babies undergoing ventilation, exchange or top-up transfusions and those needing close observation.

The "extended" role of the nursing auxiliary and the nursery nurse as documented in the course of the study is a function of the evolutionary history of neonatal care and its development. That staff employed at these levels were undertaking the care of such babies, while reflecting their experience and the needs of the service, cannot be considered appropriate or acceptable. However, many staff, particularly nursery nurses, continue to be employed in this way.

Attitudes to the Changing Role

Many D–I grade nurses expressed interest in expanding their role in neonatal care. Some wanted to take on a small number of additional tasks while others were interested in taking on a new role all together. In both cases the question of staffing was commonly raised:

> 'It would be nice to do sampling of blood gases, do our own SBR's on the unit, insert peripheral lines (venous) and intubate babies. But all these points depend on workload and staffing levels.'

'I enjoy the work in neonatal care very much. I am very interested in the role of the neonatal nurse practitioner and in the future would be willing, after training, to undertake the role. At the moment staffing levels on the unit are inadequate and until these are rectified it would be impossible to consider undertaking such a role.'

The majority of nurses who had not carried out the most common tasks wished to do so as part of their current practice: heelprick blood sampling (8 out of the 10), removal of an IV cannula (7 out of the 11) and giving IV antibiotics (104 out of 138). With the less common tasks smaller, though significant, proportions of the nurses not yet doing so, would like to expand their practice: 51% would like to be able to give drugs other than antibiotics intravenously; 63% to site IV cannulae; 71% to intubate; 40% to remove ET tubes; 63% to use a bilirubinometer and 74% to use a blood gas analyser.

Much smaller numbers of nurses would like to carry out the more invasive procedures such as performing a lumbar puncture (8%), inserting a chest drain (9%) or an umbilical arterial catheter (UAC) (16%).

Nurses Assisting Doctors

It is not surprising that so many neonatal nurses should express an interest in expanding their scope of professional practice when it is appreciated how often and how routinely nurses assist medical staff with technical procedures. Like nurses in many areas, more experienced and senior nursing staff have an active, though relatively unacknowledged role in supervising, supporting and teaching junior medical staff. They also negotiate with more senior medical staff and with other departments on behalf of SHOs, particularly those who are new in post.

'Working on SCBU we have a lot of stressful situations, but most of us dread the change over period for SHOs. Every six months we have this addition to the workload which is unnecessary as far as I am concerned. We have to constantly remind the doctors to do things which should be automatic for them, then they criticise our nursing!'

'Recently there was an uncooperative, unsupportive registrar who was unwilling to be called out and not helpful when nursing staff were unhappy with drug dosages (3 times higher than recommended) and treatment he had prescribed that was against unit policy.'

'I find the constant support and teaching of SHO's hard work – sometimes a waste of time – if they don't care about the job it's really hard to motivate them.'

Nurses working in neonatal care assist with a wide range of "medical" procedures, ranging from commonly undertaken tasks such as blood sampling and siting intravenous cannulae, through the slightly less common procedures such as lumbar puncture and exchange transfusions, to the relatively infrequent bronchial lavage or ventricular taps (Table 6.2.). Different time sampling frames can produce different pictures of activity, especially with infrequent events. Thus the results for all staff and for D–I grade nurses separately are shown for activity during the last week and during the previous three months. The frequencies shown generally reflect the technical work carried out in neonatal care and also those procedures for which nursing assistance is required.

Table 6.2 · Proportion (%) of nurses assisting with medical procedures arranged in order of frequency (Total 718 nurses, 599 D–I grade nurses)

Procedures with which nurses assisted medical staff	% D–I Nurses		% All Nurses	
	Last week	Last 3 months	Last week	Last 3 months
Blood sampling	73.5	89.8	67.7	85.1
Site IV cannula	76.3	93.0	67.7	86.5
Site IA cannula	43.1	81.8	36.6	71.2
Insert/remove UAC	30.1	83.6	25.6	71.5
Perform lumbar puncture	24.2	62.8	21.0	59.3
Insert/remove long line	19.4	58.1	16.3	55.2
Insert/remove chest drain	11.7	49.1	9.7	41.6
Bronchial lavage	9.5	20.4	7.9	17.1
SP bladder aspiration	8.5	38.1	7.5	35.1
Exchange transfusion	5.3	30.7	4.5	26.3
Insert/remove CVP	5.3	20.4	4.5	17.1
Chest aspiration	5.0	19.9	4.2	17.1
Ventricular tap	1.5	17.5	1.4	15.9
Dilution exchange	1.3	12.2	1.4	10.7
Insert/remove PD catheter	0.5	3.8	0.4	3.2

The level of seniority of the nurses assisting with some of the procedures is shown in Figures 6.6–6.9. As was expected for common procedures (for example blood sampling and siting IV cannulae) and less frequently occurring procedures (inserting or removing a UAC or a long line or performing a lumbar puncture) there are significant effects of grade (p=<0.01–<0.001). This was the case when the data are based on activity both during the last week and the last three months.

Assistance in these situations for some junior medical staff may mean being talked through a relatively unfamiliar procedure. In other situations nurses may be largely involved in preparing and setting out the equipment required, positioning, restraining and observing the baby throughout the procedure and in clearing up afterwards. Which ever of these was the case in specific instances,

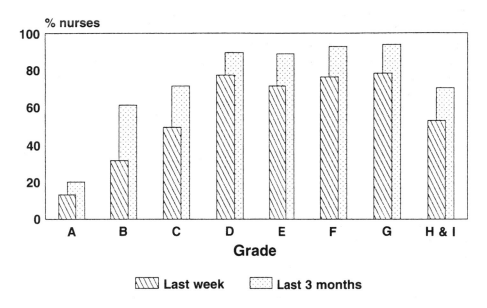

Figure 6.6 · Blood sampling procedures with which nurses at different grades gave assistance to medical staff (n=718 nurses)

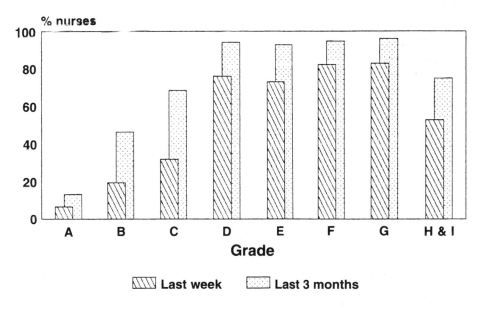

Figure 6.7 · Nurses at different grades giving assistance to medical staff in siting IV cannulae (n=718 nurses)

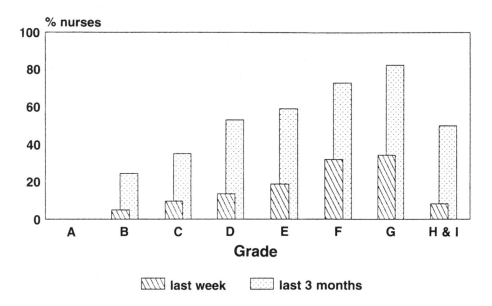

Figure 6.8 · Nurses at different grades giving assistance to medical staff in performing a lumbar puncture (n=718 nurses)

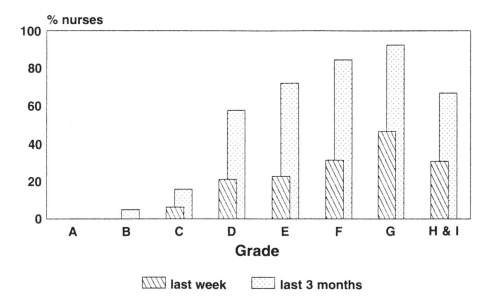

Figure 6.9 · Nurses at different grades giving assistance to medical staff in inserting or removing a UAC (n=718 nurses)

experienced nurses are clearly used as a valuable resource by medical staff, especially during procedures requiring aseptic techniques.

Unqualified nurses, as was described in the previous section, can be involved in technical areas of neonatal nursing, though at a lower frequency than staff who are registered nurses. Small numbers were involved with assisting with the siting of IA cannulae, removal or insertion of a UAC or a long line, lumbar punctures, dilution exchanges and ventricular taps. Their involvement in other procedures such as insertion or removal of chest drains and aspiration of the chest were not recorded.

The Expanding Role in Practice

It seems that some of the tasks examined have already been incorporated into the day-to-day work of nurses in neonatal care. The data collected on policy and practice appear to agree in relation to the most common tasks examined. Thus heel prick blood sampling, removal of an IV cannula and giving IV antibiotics are part of the skill base commonly expected of qualified and specialty trained nurses working in this area.

Areas of skill involving more invasive procedures, using advanced technical equipment and in which decision-making is an integral part, clearly have yet to be accepted as part of the role on a broad scale. In a small number of units, though the stated policy was for nurses not to take on such tasks, they were in fact doing so as a regular part of their work. This and the use of unqualified and untrained staff to carry out technical nursing tasks raises questions about the legal implications of these aspects of practice and the extent of liability assumed by the employing authority. To argue that untrained staff are "supervised" while carrying out the work described is ill-founded, taking into account the high levels of expertise demanded in post-basic course training and the realities of supervision. "Covering" unit staff who feel activities are within their own scope of professional practice, with or without hospital training and the use of unqualified staff as nurses working in an acute specialty like neonatal care has implications that may be serious, both for the profession and the individuals concerned.

The lower levels of practice found for H and I grades on both the common and less common tasks examined, probably reflect a reduced level of clinical involvement and more commitment in the spheres of management or teaching for some senior nurses. Changes in policy, different levels of experience and the practice of different units, may account for the frequency differences found between the relatively low proportion of nurses regularly carrying out certain tasks eg. venepuncture or removal of a chest drain and the higher proportions that have carried out these tasks at some time previously. For the nurse who has learnt new skills, moving to another unit may mean no longer being able to practice them. Local certification may be useful in the short-term to both employer and employee in financial and practical terms, but variations in policy and training, both within and between hospitals, may render this less than satisfactory in the longer term.

Differences in nursing practice between units of the kind described are likely to be a function of medical staffing and cover arrangements as well as of nursing developments. Thus, where there are fewer numbers of junior doctors or where medical cover is generally poor, nurses may have taken on duties that in other circumstances would not have been considered within their area of expertise. In some units concerns about the quality of care given to babies have led nurses to consider taking on additional tasks, despite staffing inadequacies and the absence of a planned career structure. However, the value of structured educational training programmes, adequate orientation, assessment of competence and updating of skills cannot be underestimated as required elements in preparation for professional developments of this kind (Redshaw and Harris, 1995).

The findings, supported by observations made during study visits, are based on a task-oriented approach to nursing developments in neonatal care. This approach facilitated accurate data collection and enabled a detailed profile of current practice to be constructed. However, from many perspectives the changing role of the neonatal nurse is as much a function of changing perceptions of the nursing and medical interface, as of the specific activities that may be undertaken in the role. To many neonatal nurses the changing scope of their professional practice should include elements such as nurse training, education, research and most importantly, "holistic family centred care." The evidence from the present study of nurses working in neonatal units is that there are some areas of activity which they see as part of their job and others they would like to take on, given appropriate training and recognition. However, there are some technically difficult and invasive tasks which relatively few nurses wish to encompass in their nursing role.

Choices for the Future

The boundaries and role definitions in neonatal care nursing and the interface between the work of nursing and medical staff in delivering care are changing (Harris and Redshaw, 1994; Barrett, 1995). The enhanced or expanding role of the neonatal nurse is not a universally accepted one, nor is there agreement about the additional tasks that nurses could and would be willing to take over from junior medical staff (Greenhalge, 1994; Redshaw and Harris, 1995). Some key issues, including the resource implications, will need to be addressed if professional developments in this direction are to be widely accepted and implemented and the changing skill base is to be well founded.

The effects of local training programmes varying in duration and quality need consideration. Similarly, foresight is needed concerning the consequences of initiatives by individual nurses and the medical staff responsible for teaching them in the light of the UKCC (1992 and 1994) position statements. Some neonatal nurses wish to change the boundaries, to configure their role differently and to overcome the perceived limitations of their present position, a move which has been acknowledged with the development of recognised courses for nurses in this specialty (Hall et al, 1992). Educational programmes of training and preparation for advanced practice are currently being planned and put into operation in a number of centres (Redshaw and Harris, 1995). Whether nurses learning new skills and re-defining their role will in the future continue to see themselves as nurses or as members of a new professional group, perhaps more affiliated to the medical than nursing professions, is a question for the future. Those that have a frontier perspective see the role changes discussed as simply a broadening of the scope of professional practice and a natural progression. For others, developments of this kind are at the far end of a continuum and such practitioners are perceived as metamorphosing into roles other than those associated with neonatal nurses.

References

Audit Commission (1993) Children First. HMSO, London.

Audit Commission (1995) The Doctors' Tale: Report on Medical Staffing. HMSO. London.

Barrett, G. (1995) To Extend or not to extend – that is the question. *Journal of Neonatal Nursing*, **1**, 3, 9–13.

Beresford, D. (1991) Neonatal Nurse Practitioners in Canada and Sweden. Unpublished report to Nottingham Neonatal Services.

Boxall, J. (1987) The Development of Neonatal Nurse Practitioners. Paper presented at the Neonatal Nurses Association Annual Conference, Nottingham.

Chiswick, M. and Roberton, N. (1987) Doctors and nurses in Neonatal Care: Towards integration. *Archives of Disease in Childhood*, **62**, 653–655.

Department of Health, (1989) Survey of Nurses in High Technology Care. DOH London.

Department of Health Working Group on Specialist Medical Training. (1993) Hospital Doctors: Training for the Future. Health Publications Unit, Oldham.

Drury, M., Greenfield, S., Stilwell, B. and Hull, F. (1988) A Nurse Practitioner In General Practice – Patient Perceptions and Expectations. *Journal of The Royal College of General Practitioners*. Vol.**38**, No.316, 503–505.

Greenhalge and Company (1994) The interface between junior doctors and nurses: A research study for the Department of Health.

Hale, P., Boxall, J. and Hunt, M. (1987), The role of the neonatal nurse practitioner: a viewpoint. *Archives of Disease in Childhood*, **62**, 760–1.

Hall, M., Smith, S. and Jackson, J. (1991) Neonatal Nurse Practitioners: The way forward, Origins and Development of the Wessex Initiative. "The Challenge of Caring '91" Conference, Vickers, London.

Hall, M., Smith, S., Jackson, J., Perks, E. and Walton, P. (1992) Neonatal nurse practitioners – a view from perfidious Albion?. *Archives of Disease in Childhood*, **67**:458–462.

Harper, R., Little, G. and Sia, C. (1982) The scope of nursing practice in level III neonatal intensive care units. *Paediatrics*, **70**, 875–878.

Harris, A. (1995) The Expanding Role of the Nurse in Neonatal Care. Unpublished MSc Thesis, University of Bristol.

Harris, A. and Redshaw, M. (1994) The changing role of the nurse in neonatal care: a study of current practice in England. *Journal of Advanced Nursing*, **20**, 874–880.

Harvey, D., Cooke, R. W. I. and Levitt, G. Eds. (1989) The Baby Under 1000g. Wright, London.

Herbert, F. and Little, C. (1983). Nurse Practitioner Program. University of Alberta. *Canadian Medical Association Journal*. Vol.**128**, No.11, 1311–1312.

Higginson, I. (1992) Description and preliminary evaluation of Department of Health initiatives to reduce junior doctors' hours. Report for the NHS Management Executive, Department of Health, London.

Karp, T. (1993) Neonatal nursing: Pathway to excellence or a dead end profession. Neonatal Nurses Association Conference, Nottingham.

Last, T., Self, N., Kassab, J. and Rajan, A. (1992) Extended role of the nurse in ICU. British Journal of Nursing.1,672–675.

Redshaw, M. and Harris, A. (1995) An exploratory study into the role of the advanced neonatal nurse and the educational programme of preparation. Report to the English National Board for Nursing, Midwifery and Health Visiting.

Read, S. and George, S. (1994) Nurse practitioners in accident and emergency departments. *Journal of Advanced Nursing*, **19**, 705–716.

Roberton, N. R. C. (1993) A Manual of Neonatal Intensive Care. 3rd edition. Edward Arnold, London.

Stilwell, B., Greenfield, S., Drury, M. and Hull, F. (1987). A Nurse Practitioner In General Practice. *Journal of The Royal College of General Practitioners*. Vol.**37**, No.297, 154–157.

Stock, J. and Ball, J. (1992) A Study of Nurses and Technicians in High Technology Areas. Institute of Manpower Studies. Brighton

Touche Ross Management Consultants (1994) Evaluation of Nurse Practitioner Projects. NHS Executive South Thames, London.

Trent Regional Health Authority (1995) Reduction of Junior Doctors' Hours in Trent Region, The Nursing Contribution. Trent RHA, Sheffield.

UKCC, (1992) The Scope of Professional Practice. UKCC Position Statement. London.

UKCC, (1994) The Future of Professional Practice the Councils's Standards for Education and Practice following Registration. Position Statement. London.

Chapter 7 · Nurses as Working Women

Working and Caring

As women who work, neonatal nurses are affected by the same factors that influence the lives of other working women. Many have their own families and are caring for children and other dependents while also working as nurses (Seccombe and Ball, 1992). The hours that they work, the shift worked, the need for maternity leave and for facilities related to child care are all affected by combining these two very different areas of life. Many neonatal nurses are now the main or sole wage-earner in their family and are clearly feeling the pressure:

> 'We should be paid more. It's a real worry and stress which I feel resentful about and affects my work and home life right now'

> 'If there was a wage increase I would not have to do agency work on my days off.'

> 'I worry about having a mortgage and constantly not having enough money to cover the bills.'

Though there are no immediate answers to such problems, management recognition and awareness of the concerns and worries of staff in this area is valued.

Maternity Leave

With a workforce almost exclusively made up of women (less than 1% were male), many of whom are at an active reproductive stage in their lives, pregnancy and birth are likely to be common phenomena. Yet it seems that in organising staffing, training and education, these factors are commonly not taken into account. Thus those who become pregnant and then require maternity leave may be seen as a "nuisance", "a problem" or "the last straw". They on the other hand can feel quite relieved:

> 'I was pleased to be going on maternity leave. The unit had been going through a bad patch and I felt I'd had enough.'

In the first stage of the study, data were requested on the numbers and grades of both full and part-time staff going on maternity leave in 1989 and whether they returned to work subsequently. Of the 56 units in the study, fourteen had no staff on maternity leave in 1989 and for others the number ranged from one to

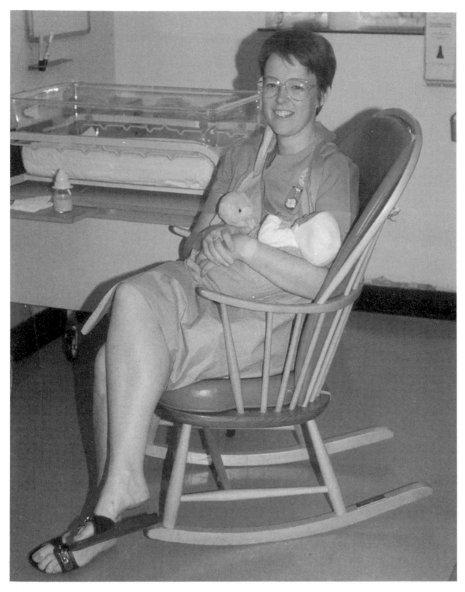

An experienced
neonatal nurse
enjoying her work in a
less intensive area of
neonatal care

nine individuals. The mean number of maternity leaves per unit for 1989 for regional units was 3.36, for sub-regional units 2.57 and for district units 1.14. Though the numbers for individual units varied, when the data were combined, the proportion of nursing staff going on maternity leave during the whole of 1989 was found to differ little between the types of unit. Over all the rate was 6%: 6% for regional units, 6.5% for sub-regional units and 5.6% for district units. In the second stage of the study individual nurses were asked about their family and if they were pregnant now. A total of 4% said they were pregnant at the time of participating in the study.

As might be expected the numbers of nurses becoming pregnant and taking maternity leave are not evenly distributed over the grades (Figure 7.1) However, in terms of proportions, the different grades taking leave match well with those employed at the different grades over all. Nurses at grade E were most likely to take maternity leave, followed by those at F and G and then D and C grades.

The returns after maternity leave taken in one year are known for 91 individuals and the relative proportions that did and did not return are shown in Figure 7.2. A relatively high rate of return (75%) was found, with 32% returning to their previous duties and 39% changing from full to part-time work. The proportion of staff returning for more than just a short period was 73% for regional units, 68% for sub-regional units and 83% for district units.

Family Commitments

Of the individual nurses in the study 83% had a partner and 54% had children. The proportions of neonatal nurses with partners and children are higher than that reported in an Royal College of Nursing survey of qualified nurses in all areas. (Seccombe and Ball, 1992). The numbers of staff with children differed significantly by unit type, with 45% of regional centre nurses having children, 59% of those in subregional units and 63% in district units (p=<0.001). Age is probably a contributor to this difference, as well as location.

Managing the care of one child while working is quite demanding, but having more than one, of differing ages and with differing needs, multiplies the demands. A total of 20% of nurses working in neonatal units had just one child, but 34% had two or more. Probably as a consequence of the need for flexible childcare, arrangements were largely dependent upon child-minding, formal and informal, or on working at weekends or nights when a partner or relative could look after the children. Workplace nurseries were present in a few hospitals, but many staff said that they were expensive and did not fit in with shift times they needed to work. A small number of holiday schemes were run for older children and those who had used them viewed such arrangements very positively.

Contrary to what might have been expected, staff with children, despite breaks in service, were more likely to have worked for longer in neonatal nursing (p=<0.001). They were also found to have taken less time off sick in the

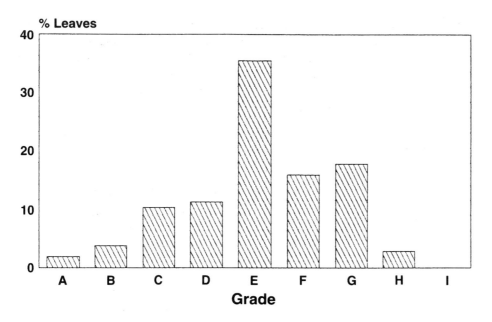

Figure 7.1 · Maternity leave taken by neonatal nurses at different grades during one year (n=56 units, 115 leaves)

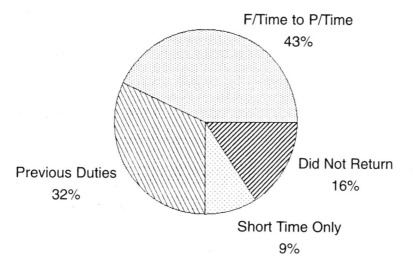

Figure 7.2 · Returns following maternity leaves taken in one year (n=56 units, 91 leaves)

previous three months ($p = <0.001$). Both of these significant relationships held when just the school age children or those below this were included. This is in contrast to the nurses studied by Seccombe and Buchan (1993) who reported that those with pre-school age children were taking more time off.

Family concerns may distract staff, but there are also important benefits when staff have families of their own:

'After having my own baby I am so much more aware of what parents can go through and feel that I am actually doing my job better.'

The problems described focused on specific occasions and issues:

'There were twenty feeds, all different and no one to help. I only work part time. I had to work over and my two children sat on the doorstep waiting for me.'

'I received a phone call at work from my partner; my son aged two years had an accident. Although he sustained minor injuries, because of staff shortages I was not allowed to go home. All that shift I did not function as well as usual and forgot to do minor things. I could quite easily have been negligent.'

'I am working two night shifts per week and looking after two small children leading to extreme tiredness, irritability, and difficulty coping at work. It is very stressful juggling childcare and problems when children are ill.'

'I was upset having specially requested and been refused Christmas off as a single parent of four children – nobody is allowed it off.'

The difficulties that many neonatal nurses experience adjusting after a break in their careers may work against them returning to neonatal care:

'I was away from nursing for 14 years bringing up my family. I left the SCBU in this hospital and came back to it again. I felt as though I had stepped onto a strange planet where everything had changed, including the language. The babies, equipment, terminology and technology had altered beyond my comprehension while I was away'.

'I started on a new unit after a 12 month break during which time I moved house and had a baby. The management was expecting a lot from me, while I was feeling inadequate – from "just a housewife" to a staff nurse in a busy understaffed unit.'

However, the maturity, broader skill base and motivation of this group are worth investing in, but until training and update schemes adjust to their needs, it seems that full re-entry into the workforce may be limited.

Part-Time Nurses

Part-time nursing, often during unsocial hours, may be an essential way of contributing to the family income, while still being able to care for dependents. Combining part-time working and caring for children is not easy and in some cases is not supported by management policies. For example, returns to work can be influenced in this way. In only 39 (70%) of the 56 first phase study units were staff who were changing from full to part-time work allowed to return to work at the same grade. In some units the rules were applied differently for different grades. The apparent arbitrariness of such rules and differences in attitude were what seemed to upset the individual nurses concerned:

> 'I am a qualified and experienced neonatal nurse working three days a week, but because I work part-time after returning from maternity leave, I cannot be given the grade I would be entitled to if I worked full-time.'

> 'I work part-time as I have a small son. "F" grade posts came up on the unit. I was told I could apply if I could increase my hours to 30+ per week. I was also told I would not be considered favourably as they were expecting me to have another child soon! I did not apply, and instead applied for an "F" grade at another hospital on 20 hours a week.'

> 'I am a part-time member of the night staff because of family commitments. I feel that no attempt is made to meet my needs in this dual role.'

> 'Being a part-time member of the night staff I find myself under-valued by others. In terms of my career, at times I feel frustrated due to the restrictions that having a young family places on me.'

For some individuals working part-time provides a relief and a diversion as well as a financial benefit, while full-time work would be experienced as too stressful:

> 'I am very thankful to have such an enjoyable job. My colleagues are very friendly to work with and it's a pleasure to go to work most of the time. Working two days per week and looking after my family is a good balance for me.'

> 'It can be hard at times, managing a job and family and being pregnant, but it's a welcome outlet at times.'

Details of part-time working were collected at the same point as grade information. In the 56 units 43% of the workforce were nurses working less than full-time hours. The proportion of part-time staff employed differed significantly depending on the type of unit: regional units had the least (35%); subregional had more (44%) and district units had the largest numbers (51%). Part-time working was also found to differ significantly according to grade. The relative proportions of full and part-time staff at the different grades is shown in Figure 7.3. From this it is clear that at the lower end of the scale the staff are predominantly part-time, while at the upper end part-time working is rare. The actual proportions as part of the whole workforce are shown by unit type in Figure 7.4.

The data collected on individual nurses participating in the study confirmed these findings: overall the proportion of staff working part-time was 47%; 40% of nurses working in regional centres did so on a part-time basis; 48% of those in subregional units and 52% in district units. The relative proportions of part and full-time staff at different grades were also similar to those found in the first stage of the project.

Part-time working seems to be more common in neonatal care than in nursing generally, as across the whole profession the comparable figure reported by Seccombe and Ball (1992) is 32%. Whether the difference is a function of the age structure of the workforce in the specialty, of the staffing problems described in Chapters 3 and 4, or of other factors is open to debate. What is meant by "part-time" working appears to be anything less than full-time work at 37.5 hours per week. In fact the contract hours for individual nurses ranged from less than ten to 40 hours per week. Though overall 57% of the workforce have contracts that are 35 hours per week or more, there are substantial numbers of staff working a wide range of hours (Figure 7.5.). Different patterns of use by the different types of unit are shown in Figure 7.6.

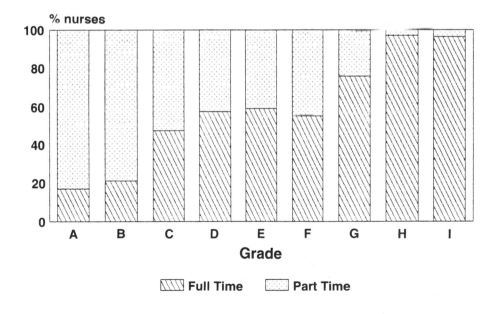

Figure 7.3 · Proportion of nurses working full and part-time at different grades (n=56 units, 1890 nurses)

REGIONAL UNITS

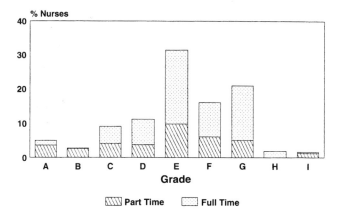

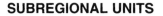

SUBREGIONAL UNITS

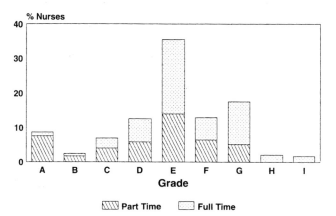

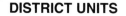

DISTRICT UNITS

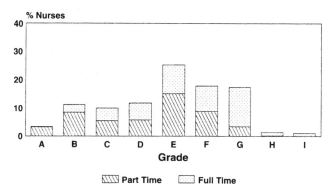

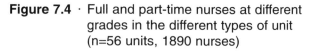

Figure 7.4 · Full and part-time nurses at different grades in the different types of unit (n=56 units, 1890 nurses)

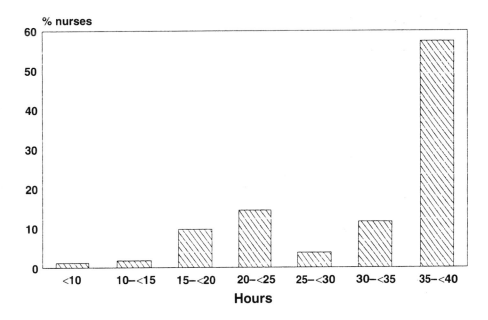

Figure 7.5 · Contract hours worked by neonatal nurses (n=24 units)

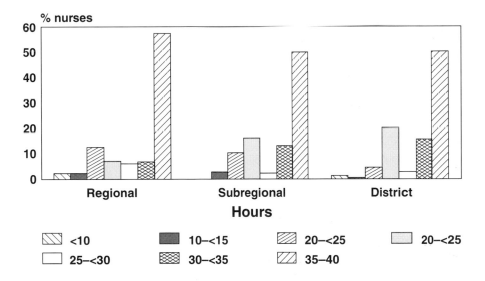

Figure 7.6 · Contract hours worked by neonatal nurses in different types of unit (n=24 units)

The variation in contract hours, though possibly giving neonatal nurses flexibility about the hours worked, is also likely to be a reflection of the staffing and skill mix problems and shortages discussed in Chapters 3 and 4.

Senior nursing management seems to vary in its attitude to part-time neonatal nurses. In a few units there is a policy of not employing any part-time staff and yet for most units, they are a vital part of the team. One of the needs expressed by working women, particularly those with children, is for flexibility in the work situation. Working part-time, at unsocial hours is for some neonatal nurses the way to have that flexibility. The large contribution made by nurses working less than full-time hours is evident as are the lower turnover rates for this group (Gray and Phillips, 1994). It would seem that retention could be enhanced further, at least in some units, if this issue were addressed more fairly.

Working on the Night Shift

The costs and benefits of working a shift system and conflicts related to the organisation of domestic and social life are recognised. A recent study (Barton et al, 1993a; Barton et al, 1993b) forms part of a larger research project aimed at trying to identify shift systems or features of shift systems which are likely to have the least detrimental effects on the health and wellbeing of individual nurses. Some of the inevitable problems experienced by those engaged in shift work are biological in nature, centering on the disturbance of physiological rhythms, including the sleep-wake cycle. There may also be impairment of physical and psychological health and social and domestic disruption. Many of these shift work associated problems are believed to occur when there is a mismatch between the internal "body clock" and external cues.

In recent years there has been a movement away from very rigid shift systems towards those which are more flexible in nature. The practice of "flexible rostering" can give the individuals involved more control over the organisation of their work and it is also thought to have positive benefits for the hospital concerned (Elliot, 1989). These include opportunities to increase the numbers of staff during peak hours of the day, attempts to improve communication among personnel during hand-overs and to decrease absenteeism and overtime.

In the past many women with young children have chosen to work on the night shift because the shifts are longer and they need to work fewer shifts to complete full-time hours. Some have then continued to work at night, though the family need is no longer there. The established nurses with "nights only" contracts valued these highly:

> 'Permanent night duty is not really thought a good thing but I have worked many years here and enjoyed seeing the development of neonatal intensive care from almost its start. I have usually felt it a worthwhile job and been happy and felt appreciated.'

Such contracts are gradually becoming less common as new staff are taken on with some rotation to days written into their working agreements. However, nurses working on the night shift were clear about the benefits and the attitudes towards them as night shift staff:

> 'I have just started on nights and find it's more relaxing than on the day shift. You have no parents, its just you and the babies, though the longer shifts are very tiring.'

> 'On night duty we work as a closely-knit team and give help and support to each other.'

> 'As part of the night shift, I am fed up with people assuming that all I do is knit all night and that I appear to be completely brain dead. The truth is that the atmosphere is far better on nights, but the workload in terms of quantity and quality is exactly the same.'

> 'I have been on night duty for the last 3 months. The night staff are all experienced and work well together and there is little change in staff. On day duty there are frequent changes, many staff are inexperienced and need a lot of supervision, there is less team work and they find it difficult to work together.'

Of the 718 individual nurses studied, 28% just worked on the night shift and as was shown in Chapter 4 on skill mix, these tended to be at the lower and cheaper end of the scale. The need is thus even greater for this group to be included in update and inservice training. In some instances the need for update has been denied or resisted, but many nurses themselves recognise the problem:

> 'Because I only work one night a week, things change quite a bit and I find it difficult to cope with ringing up the radiologist etc. I have forgotten how to do it or can't find the number. Also I don't like helping with drips as I never know when to put pressure on or let go. Because I have been here a long time I feel a fool to ask.'

In contrast to many shiftwork research findings and changing management policy, two recent studies of nurses have produced results which add support to the case for the adoption of a permanent night shift, emphasising the benefits for the health and wellbeing of individual nurses (Verhaegen et al 1987; Barton and Folkard, 1991). The physical and psychological effects of nurses working different shifts are discussed in the chapter which follows.

Working Women as Professional Carers

As an essentially female workforce the needs of this group of nurses could be better addressed in a wider variety of ways. One way of improving the staffing levels and increasing retention may be to increase flexibility over the hours worked, though at the lowest levels keeping skills up to date is a problem which must be dealt with at the same time. The need for compassionate and "carers leave" for those with children and other dependents must be reviewed and less inflexible policies developed and implemented. For example the negotiation of temporary reductions in hours, may enable an individual to continue working through a time of family crisis, rather than being lost to the workforce all together. The requirements for antenatal care and maternity leave should be adequately addressed in calculating staffing and establishment figures. The role of the workplace in facilitating the provision of child care demands more serious attention and the implications of change to a twelve hour shift system for women with dependents considered.

The need for more flexibility for women workers in the health service, with regard to both working arrangements and training schemes has been recognised and made explicit in the Opportunity 2000 document (DOH/NHSME, 1993). Modularisation of courses, longer time scales for completion of courses and the development of distance learning packages may assist in the area of education. However, achievement of the goal of more flexible working arrangements through the implementation of innovative working practices will probably be dependent upon the willingness of nurses and NHS Trusts to experiment in this area.

Whatever schemes are tried it is clear that there are benefits in having at least part of the workforce in neonatal care made up of individuals with direct experience in caring for their own families. With the moves towards more family centred care, the ability to understand and empathise with the experiences of the client group and their families is a valuable asset in those undertaking their care. As one of the most stable parts of the workforce in neonatal care the nurses who have dependents and who work part-time, often at night, are a resource whose needs and value are worth recognising.

References

Barton, J. and Folkard, S. (1991) The response of day and night nurses to their work schedules. *J. Occupational Psychology*, **64**. 207–218.

Barton, J., Smith, I., Totterdell, P. A., Spelton, E. R. and Folkard, S. (1993a) Does individual choice determine shift system acceptability? *Ergonomics*, **36**, 93–99.

Barton, J., Spelton, E. R., Smith, I., Totterdell, P. A., and Folkard, S. (1993b) A classification of nursing and midwifery shift systems. *Int. J. Nursing Studies*, **30**, 65–80.

Elliot, T. L. (1989) Cost analysis of alternative scheduling. *Nursing Management*, **20**, 42–47.

Gray, A. M. and Phillips, V. L.(1994) Turnover, age and length of services: A comparison of nurses and other staff in the National Health Service. *Journal of Advanced Nursing*, **19**, 819–827.

Hingley, P. and Cooper, C. (1989) Stress and the Nurse Manager. Wiley, Chichester.

Opportunity 2000 (1992) NHSME. London.

Seccombe, I. and Ball, J. (1992) Motivation, Morale and Mobility. IMS Report No 233, IMS Brighton.

Seccombe, I. and Buchan, J. (1993) Absent Nurses: The costs and Consequences. IMS Report No 250, IMS, Brighton.

Verhaegen, P., Cober, R., DeSmedt, M., Dirkx, J., Kerstens, J. and Van Daele, P. (1987) The adaptation of night nurses to different work schedules. *Ergonomics*, **30**, 1301–1309.

Chapter 8 · Physical Health and Psychological Wellbeing

Working in Neonatal Care

The health of an individual is affected by many different factors, one of which is the working environment. Neonatal nurses do shift work, inside, under artificial lighting, in relatively high temperatures, exposed to illness and infection and the stresses of coping with the needs of babies, parents and colleagues. It has been suggested that personnel working in intensive care settings are particularly susceptible to emotional stress (Strickland et al, 1980; Marshall and Kasman, 1980; Astbury and Yu, 1982). Many of the nursing staff working with preterm infants, babies with congenital abnormalities and babies with other problems are at a stage in their lives when they themselves may be having children or considering doing so. This may result in greater empathy with the small patients and families but it may also complicate the responses and adjustments made in dealing with what is an abnormal situation.

Neonatal care is a rapidly changing specialty and the demands on neonatal nurses in terms of technical and interpersonal skills are high. Increasing interest has been expressed in the way staff function in this context (Gray-Toft and Anderson, 1981; Bender, 1981; Walker, 1982) but relatively few empirical studies have been carried out on the work experiences, effects on health and wellbeing and coping strategies of staff choosing to work in this kind of environment (Jacobson, 1978; 1983).

The focus in this chapter is on how different individual nurses respond to working in neonatal care and what strategies they have for maintaining their health and wellbeing while working there. In order to develop a more complete description of the neonatal unit as a working environment a wide range of physical health and psychological factors were investigated. Measures of weight and height were included, as were recent illnesses, smoking, exercise, anxiety, social support and perceived sources of stress and concern.

One of the most obvious ways to look for the evidence of stress in the work situation is to examine the records for sickness and absenteeism. Data on sick leave were collected from the 56 units in the first stage of the study and returned from 718 individual nurses in the second stage. Individual information was also collected on a wide range of other topics related to health during this second stage. The findings on these different areas will be presented separately.

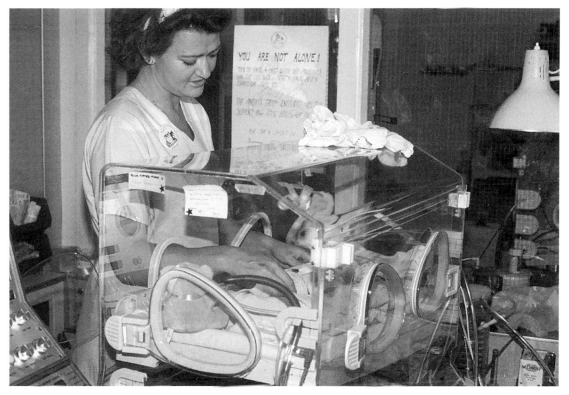

*A nurse caring for a
very low birth weight
baby in the intensive
care area of the unit*

General Health

Individual nurses from the 24 units participating in the second stage of the study were asked about their current general health. The majority described themselves as fit and well (63%), a third said they were mostly well and healthy (33%), but a small proportion were rarely well or often ill (4%). The individual nurses were also asked if they ate a healthy diet: 14% always did so, 76% mostly did but 10% did so only occasionally or not at all. Data on the heights and weights of individual nurses were requested and excluding those who were pregnant, 676 nurses provided both items of information. The weights ranged from 39 to 114 kilos (mean 62 Kg and median 60 Kg) and the heights from 1.45 metres to 1.73 metres (mean 1.63 m., median 1.62 m.). The height and weight measurements were combined to produce five appropriate height for weight categories (Metropolitan Life, 1983). The two extremes were examined and it was concluded that 13% could be categorised as markedly underweight for their height and 18% were markedly overweight. However, using a body mass index (Blaxter, 1990) the numbers of neonatal nursing staff that were obese and underweight were found to be little different from a general population of non-manual working women.

The nurse subjects were also asked about smoking, alcohol and caffeine consumption. A total of 14% were smokers: 46% of whom smoked less than 10 cigarettes per day; 51% smoked 10–20 cigarettes; and 3% smoked more than this. The overall figure for smoking was less than the 33% reported for the general population, and the 27% reported for nurse managers and ward sisters (Hingley and Cooper, 1986). The numbers of cigarettes smoked by those who did so, were less than those reported by the same authors. Most neonatal nurses (64%) drank alcohol only rarely or not at all, 30% did so once or twice a week, 10% drank between 3 and 6 times per week and 1% drank every day. Comparisons with other groups on the consumption of alcohol are difficult to make, but if the highest categories are combined it seems that neonatal nurses behave similarly to the managers and ward sisters studied by Hingley and Cooper (1986). They concluded that nurses were drinking no more than women in the general population. A small proportion of nurses had no caffeinated drinks at all (6%), the majority (71%) drank up to six cups per day, but 22% drank more than this. Though the consumption of all of these did not appear to differ according to the type of unit worked in, there may perhaps be concern about the effects on those drinking alcohol in the more frequent categories.

Sickness

Neonatal nurses may see themselves as mainly healthy, but many take time off sick. Data were requested on the days taken as sick leave for each of the fifty-six study units during 1989. Documentation of sickness figures does not appear to be uniformly carried out. However, the number of days of recorded sick leave taken in the whole of 1989 was returned from forty-two of the fifty-six units. That half the regional units were unable to provide these data may reflect the difficulty of maintaining records on the large numbers of staff involved, or possibly a reluctance to disclose them. Computerisation may assist with the routine collection of these kind of data.

In order to take account of the variable size of units, these data were examined in terms of sickness rate. This was calculated in two ways, first as the numbers of days taken per whole time equivalent and secondly as the number of days taken per nurse employed by grade. This is because in some instances the WTE establishment figure is less reliable as it takes no account of vacancies and in some cases is below even the lowest recommended levels. The 1990 establishment figures in WTEs and the number of nurses employed by grade at the time of the study in 1990 were used for these calculations. Details of the sickness figures collected are given in Table 8.1. Overall the sickness rates for all the units combined were 10.2 days per WTE and 9.2 days per nurse employed and there was a significant effect of unit type on the sickness rate calculated in both ways.

Table 8.1 · Annual sickness rates in different types of unit (n=42 units)

	Unit Type		
	Regional (n=7)	Sub-regional (n=12)	District (n=23)
Average days sick per unit	587.29	404.42	165.71
Days off sick per WTE	9.77	11.09	9.62
Days off sick per nurse employed	10.07	9.91	7.52

The data discussed above were reported by unit managers or senior nurses and were for each unit as a whole. In order to obtain more detailed information, in the second stage individual nurses were asked about the sick leave they had taken in the previous three months, both with and without a sick note. The data presented in Table 8.2. show that 28% of the nursing staff took notified sick leave during this time and that 17% also took un-notified sick leave.

For both notified and un-notified sick leave the amounts of time taken for each nurse who was sick and the mean leave taken per nurse employed were highest for the regional centres, followed by the district units and then the subregional units. If the sick leave taken in a year for these individuals is assumed to be four times the amount of sick leave taken in three months, then overall the rate per nurse employed, at 8.96 days is very close to the 9.2 days obtained from the data collected from the unit managers. However, the actual rate is higher for the largest units, though in contrast to the first stage findings, the district units rank next highest rather than the subregional units. The difference between these data may reflect changes over the two years between data collection points or possibly greater accuracy in the data obtained after visits to the units.

That notified sick leave was five times as frequent as un-notified leave could indicate that most neonatal nurses are not just calling in at the last moment, taking what could be called "stress days", or else that most are expected to provide certificates, no matter how short a time they are off sick. However, it is of interest to note that in comparison with the profession as a whole, neonatal nurses seem to be taking less time off sick. The survey by Seccombe and Ball (1993) showed a wide range in reported absence levels, averaging around 14 days for qualified nurses and 17 days for nursing auxiliaries. A similar finding was reported by the Audit Commission (1994) on sickness in fourteen different hospital and community trusts. Only two of the fourteen trusts had an average

Table 8.2a · Amount of time taken as notified sick leave during previous 3 months (n=718 nurses)

Notified sick leave	Regional	Sub-regional	District	Overall
%	28.91	25.64	29.26	28.17
Mean leave (days)	8.33	4.12	6.40	6.65
Median (days)	3	2	3	3
Range (days)	1–56	1–30	1–52	1–56
Per nurse employed (days)	2.41	1.06	1.87	1.87

Table 8.2b · Amount of time taken as un-notified sick leave during previous 3 months (n=718 nurses)

Un-notified sick leave	Regional	Sub-regional	District	Overall
%	18.71	13.85	17.46	16.99
Mean leave (days)	2.18	1.85	2.35	2.16
Median (days)	2	2	1	2
Range (days)	1–7	1–4	1–4	1–7
Per nurse employed (days)	0.41	0.26	0.41	0.37

rate of less than 10 days per year for qualified nurses and six had average rates of above 15 days per year.

Reasons for Sick Leave

Nurses were also asked about hospital stays in the last year. Of the whole population 15% had been admitted to hospital and stays ranged from 1–70 days (with a mean of 4.18 days and median of 2 days). The reasons for admission are shown in Figure 8.1. and included obstetric cases, gynaecological problems, surgery, and observation or investigations.

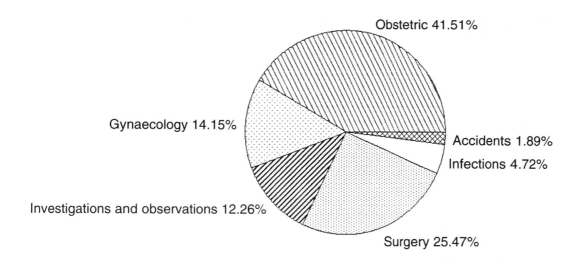

Figure 8.1 · Reasons for admission to hospital (n=24 units, 111 nurses)

These data and those on sick leave as a whole indicate that most nurses are off for relatively short periods of time, but there is also a small group who are off work for quite extended periods. There are also nurses who work despite being unwell. Individual nurses were given a check list of illnesses and conditions and asked to indicate which they had suffered from in the last year and which had caused them to take time off work. The items on the list were selected to include common illnesses, but also conditions that have been reported in the health literature as potentially stress-related (Hingley and Cooper, 1986).

The proportions of nurses experiencing and taking time off for the most common conditions is shown in Figure 8.2a. Less common but significant conditions are listed in Figure 8.2b. From these figures it can be seen that the most frequently occurring problems are coughs and colds, headaches and backaches from which 77%, 67% and 35% of neonatal nurses suffered. A total of 21% reported that they suffered from anxiety, 10% from depression, 24% from indigestion and 10% from eczema or psoriasis. The effects of work largely carried out while standing in a hot, enclosed, stressful environment may to some extent explain these data. Many nurses clearly continued to work with a variety of health problems, some of which may have been exacerbated by continuing to do so, others which may have put babies and other staff at risk.

Overall, the level of most types of medication taken in the last year was relatively low: sleeping pills were at times taken by 8% of nurses, tranquillisers by 1%, anti-depressants by 2%, and antacids 5%. In contrast to these incidences, 67% of nurses had taken painkillers and 41% had taken one or more courses of antibiotics.

Sickness requiring time off was greatest amongst those nurses working full-time (p=<0.05) and those who had no children (p=<0.01). The total illnesses

ILLNESSES AND CONDITIONS

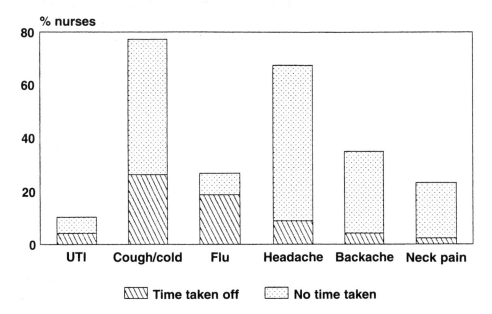

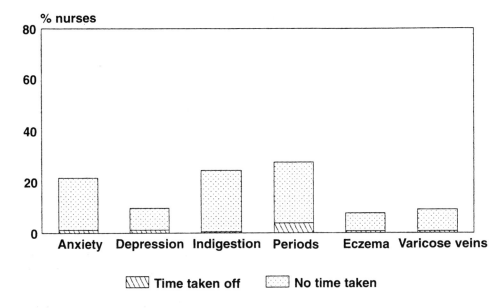

Figure 8.2 · Illnesses and conditions experienced in the last year, with and without time off (n=718 nurses)

experienced in the last year and the sick leave per nurse were higher in regional and district units than subregional units ((p=<0.02), p=<0.05). It also varied according to age (p=<0.001) with the nurses aged 20–29 and then those aged 50–59 taking most time off and the oldest age group at 60 or more years, taking least.

Physical and Psychological Factors

Relationships between illnesses experienced, time taken as sick leave and aspects of the working environment are complex. That a large amount of time is taken as sick leave, and considerable numbers of staff are experiencing anxiety and depression, as well as colds, flu and other infections requiring treatment, is of some concern. The boundary between physical and psychological wellbeing is a narrow and variable one for most individuals and for those working under the stressful conditions of neonatal care the difference is likely to be more difficult to define.

Neonatal units care for babies that cannot be cared for in other parts of the hospital or at home. The major responsibility for the performance of this primary task lies with the nursing staff who must provide continuous care for these babies, day and night, all year round. Neonatal nurses, like the hospital nurses studied by Menzies (1970), bear "the full, immediate and concentrated impact of stresses arising directly or indirectly from patient care". They are confronted with the threat and reality of death in ways that few lay people experience and their work situation can arouse strong feelings in them as individuals and professionals. The direct impact of looking after small, often sick babies is intensified by facing and dealing with psychological stress in other people, including work colleagues and parents. Organisational problems can compound the effect: the threat of crisis, operational breakdown and radical change, all have consequences for the individual.

Mental Health

The General Health Questionnaire is the most widely applied measure of psychiatric disturbance in the UK (Goldberg, 1978; Goldberg and Williams, 1988). It is a screening questionnaire assessing present state, used for detecting psychiatric disorder, particularly anxiety and depression, rather than long-term chronic problems.

As part of the nurses' package in the pilot study the GHQ 28-item version was used, but for practical purposes, with the large amount of data to be collected it was decided to use the shorter GHQ12 for the main study group. This short version is reported to be as efficient as longer versions as a case detector (Goldberg and Williams, 1988; Bowling, 1991). In choosing this extensively used instrument it was hoped to compare the study data on this aspect of health with that from research on other groups (Bowling, 1991; Spelton et al, 1993).

Of the whole sample of nurses 715 completed the GHQ 12. If the threshold is set at scores of 2 or more, 44% of this population were above this level. With a higher threshold of 3 or more the proportion above the threshold is 33%. As 21% and 10% of neonatal nurses had reported themselves directly as suffering from anxiety and depression, then it is perhaps not surprising that the proportions scoring above the thresholds should be as large as were found. The GHQ12 scores for nurses working in the different types of unit are shown in Table 8.3.

Table 8.3 · General Health Questionnaire scores for nurses working in different types of unit (n=715 nurses)

	Unit Type		
	Regional	Subregional	District
Mean Score	2.53	2.03	2.12
Median Score	1	1	1
SD	3.05	2.93	3.03
Range	0–12	0–12	0–12
% 2 or <	48	40	42
% 3 or <	39	28	31

As the subject sample consisted almost entirely of women, the majority of whom were of child-bearing age, a check was made on those who had recently been pregnant or had a baby in the last year. No significant differences in the rates of depression and anxiety were found between these groups and the rest of the study population. However, it is of interest to compare the 10% depression among neonatal nurses with rates recorded among post-natal mothers. The prevalence rate for depression at any time in the first year after childbirth is in the order of 10–20% (Watson el al, 1984; Cooper et al, 1988) and among post-natal mothers a perceived lack of social and emotional support from a partner is strongly associated with depression at this time (Kumar and Robson, 1984; O'Hara et al, 1986). These kind of possible links with depression and psychological wellbeing more generally were explored among the study group of neonatal nurses as part of the multivariate analyses described later in the chapter.

The differences between the nurses working in regional, subregional and district units approached significance, but there were more statistically significant relationships with other variables: age ($p=<0.02$), full or part-time work (p=<0.002), type of shift (p=<0.001), presence or absence of partner (p=<0.05), and not having children (p=<0.02) This means that those with higher GHQ scores were more likely to be in the younger (20–29 years, 30–39 years) and oldest (60+ years) age groups; more often working full-time; more often working a rotating shift and less likely to have a partner or children. Variables that were not found to be associated were the grade at which they were employed, being qualified in the specialty, or having family living locally. However, the GHQ scores were significantly correlated with the total time taken for sick leave in the last three months (r=.24) and with the scores on the instrument used to measure occupational stress (r=.39) (The Nurse Stress Index, Harris et al, 1988) (p=<0.001).

Data collected on ward-based and community psychiatric nurses found the latter to have a significantly higher threshold, with 41% scoring five or more on the GHQ28 (Brown et al, 1994). In a study of occupational stress in high dependency nursing using the GHQ28 Tyler and Ellison (1994), as in the present study, found a relationship with the presence of a partner and a correlation with the NSI scores. Using the GHQ12 at three different time points in a study of the impact of night work on the psychological wellbeing of student nurses, Bohle and Tilley (1989) used a Likert style scoring system with each of the twelve items scoring from 0–3. Mean scores increased with the introduction of shift work and the students whose shifts included night working scored higher, indicating that the introduction of night work had a significant negative impact on wellbeing.

Comparison of Likert type GHQ12 scores on a general population of hospital nurses (Spelton et al, 1993) with the nurses working in neonatal care shows a difference, with the female shiftwork study respondents on average having slightly higher scores than the neonatal nurses studied. Perhaps of more interest is the finding that those working permanently on the night shift had significantly lower GHQ scores than their counterparts rotating between shifts. Age and the total hours worked also appear to be important factors, but relatively little relationship was found by Spelton and her colleagues (1993) between psychological symptoms and the type of ward, dependency of patients cared for, or with grade of clinical post or title.

Coping and Social Support

In addition to reporting illnesses and symptoms, all the nurses in the study were asked about how they felt at the end of a shift. Table 8.4. shows the way different proportions of nurses commonly felt at the end of a working day.

Strategies for coping with stress of all types vary. Among nurses of all types experiencing occupational stress these have included direct action or problem-solving behaviour, trying to unwind and put things in perspective, expressing feelings or frustration, keeping the problem to yourself, accepting the job as it is and trying not to let it get to you (Dewe, 1987). Among nurses working in

Table 8.4 · How nurses working in neonatal care commonly feel at the end of a shift (n=718 nurses)

Adjectives used by nursing staff		
	73%	Exhausted
	49%	Relieved
	31%	Strained
% Often or usually	25%	Tense
	15%	Low
	12%	Angry
	11%	Inadequate
	10%	Emotional

neonatal intensive care in the United States, Jacobson (1983) found that focusing on family, friends or hobbies was the most common strategy, followed by building on one's own competence, changing the approach to the job, taking breaks or vacations, responding emotionally and by changing jobs.

In the neonatal units studied in England, nurses seem to behave similarly. As was mentioned previously some smoke, drink alcohol or consume large amounts of caffeine and some may have been using food or control of the consumption of food as coping mechanisms. Another way of coping is to turn to outside activities. Quite a number of nurses took exercise in the form of cycling, riding, jogging or brisk walking on a daily basis (20%) and a further 29% did so at least once a week. A total of 13% did aerobics, gym or keep-fit at least once a week or more. Less vigorous recreational activity was also reported with 5% doing yoga or meditation and 35% using art, craft or music one or more times per week. Other interests are important and many neonatal nurses have a pet (54%). Cats were most common, followed by dogs, though a wide range of other mammals including horses, guinea pigs and rabbits were reported. Birds, fish and invertebrates were also kept as pets.

The importance of personality traits as an intervening variable in the stress equation was emphasised by Cooper and Marshall (1976). Psychometric and behavioural individual differences data play a crucial role in the person-environment fit and the manifestation of stress and stress related disease. "Type A coronary prone behaviour" is made up of a cluster of traits and is characterised by extremes of competitiveness, striving for achievement, impatience, aggressiveness and a low tolerance of stress. The 14 item scale (Bortner and Rosenman, 1967) used by Hingley and Cooper (1986) in their study of nurse managers, was also used in the present study. Scores can range from 14 to 154, with higher scores being indicative of Type A behaviour. Four categories are classified along the continuum; Type A1 (108–154), Type A2 (93–107), Type B3 (64–92) and Type B4 (14–53).

The neonatal nurses in the present study differ from the nurses managers studied by Hingley and Cooper and the general population (Davidson and

Cooper, 1983) (Table 8.5.). Both the whole population (n=709) and the G, H and I grade nurses alone (n=164) show a distribution that is markedly different, being clearly skewed towards the Type B traits. As high occupational status is thought to be related to Type A behaviour, particularly among working women in the 40–59 age range (Waldron, 1978) this is a slightly surprising finding. The higher proportion of part-time nurses working in neonatal care and changing economic circumstances, resulting in many non-career nurses returning or continuing to work may have contributed to this difference. It may also be that the nature of work in neonatal care itself has a selective effect and those who continue to be able to work in the specialty are different in this respect.

Table 8.5 · Distribution of Type A behaviour scores of neonatal nurses and other groups (%) (n=718 nurses)

	Type			
	A1	A2	B3	B4
General Population (Davidson and Cooper, 1983)	10	40	40	10
Female Executives (Davidson and Cooper, 1980)	21.5	40.0	38.5	0.0
Nurse Managers (Hingley and Cooper, 1986)	21.2	34.0	41.4	3.1
Neonatal Nurses (All)	0.9	8.6	79.6	11.0
Neonatal Nurses (G, H and I grades only)	1.2	10.4	80.5	7.9

Another key factor that is thought to be a moderating influence in the experience and effects of stress is that of social support (Cooper and Payne, 1978). It was felt that with a profession in which a great deal is demanded in the way of giving support to others, it was important to consider the sources of support available to neonatal nurses. Demographic questions, some of which were referred to in Chapter 7, had been asked as part of the study and these revealed that 9% of neonatal nurses were living alone, 5% with their parents and 9% with friends or in a nurses home. A total of 83% had partners, 54% had children and 60% had family living locally. When asked about their own sources of social support the study nurses ranked their partner first, followed by friends, family, work colleagues and then mentioned others including their dog, God and a counsellor. A small number of nurses reported having only one (5%) or no (2%) close friends. The responses to being asked about the

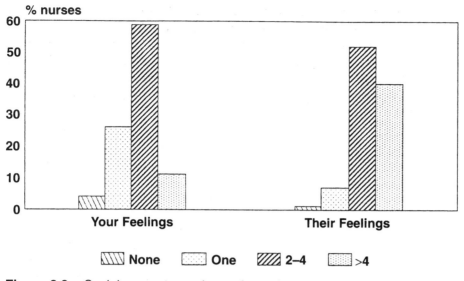

Figure 8.3 · Social support: numbers of people nurses talked to about personal problems and feelings (n=718)

numbers of people that they could talk to about their personal problems and feelings and the numbers of people that talked to them in the same way are shown in Figure 8.3. In terms of family and friends neonatal nurses seem to be giving more social support than they receive and this is in addition to their work in caring for the parents of babies who are looked after in neonatal care. Self selection for working in a caring profession may be a factor here. However, it is also possible that for some nurses with promotion and changes of job and location, social isolation is increased.

Mechanisms for addressing work issues formally seem to be limited: discussing difficulties at work was found to take place formally for only 24% of nurses, though 87% of nurses did so informally. Being able to discuss work difficulties at home and with friends were essential elements in most individuals' coping mechanisms, though for those with few friends or living alone the situation may be more bleak.

Stress in Neonatal Nursing

There are many different explanations of stress which can be conceptualised in a variety of ways. For the purposes of the current research an interactionist approach is taken in which stress arises as a function of an individual interacting with the environment (Lazarus, 1976). A transactional view of the person and his or her environment as elements in a dynamic system, involves a balance between demands, both internal and external and the capacity to meet those demands. The intensity of the stress experienced is determined by how well an individual feels he or she can deal with problems identified. If he has confidence in his coping abilities, the effects are minimised, whereas if a person is unsure of these, they are likely to feel helpless and overwhelmed.

Stress is a common feature of many work situations, particularly for those working in hospital environments (Parkes, 1985, Payne and Firth-Cozens, 1987). Among the potential stressors in the workplace are the nature of relationships with work colleagues, role conflict, role ambiguity, workload and the work environment. In some work situations, such as the neonatal unit, where failure to meet demands has important consequences, the effects of such an imbalance between demands and response capability are likely to be heightened. Potential stressors produce different reactions in different people. "Stress is not only what happens to you, but how you take what happens to you" (Lachman, 1983). In interacting with the working environment individual differences, such as personality, demographic factors, physical characteristics, past history, experience and motivation may function as mediating variables. In the present study the focus was mostly on the measures that could show how stressed neonatal nurses are and the sources of stress. Less emphasis was placed on coping strategies, though some mediating variables are examined.

The Nurse Stress Index (Harris et al, 1988) was selected for use in this study as a means of assessing occupational stress in the neonatal unit environment. It was designed as an instrument to pinpoint and measure the main sources of stress in the day-to-day work of nurses and had recently been used with a wide range of nurses, including nurse managers (Hingley and Cooper, 1986). The index is constructed with six sub-scales: managing the workload (MW1 and MW2); organisational support and involvement (OSI); dealing with patients and relatives (DPR); home and work conflict (HWC) and confidence and competence in role (CCR). Interpretation of results is based on reference to norms provided for nurses working in rural or urban settings. The latter were used for comparison in Table 8.6.

Table 8.6 · A comparison of total and sub-scale scores on the Nurse Stress Index for the study nurses and those reported by Harris et al (1988)

Urban Hospital Nurses	Nurse stress index subscales						
	MW1	MW2	OSI	DPR	HWC	CCR	Total
Mean	12.5	12.0	12.0	10.2	7.5	10.0	64.2
SD	4.3	3.9	4.7	3.8	2.8	3.4	16.7
Neonatal Nurses							
Mean	12.3	12.6	13.8	12.2	9.5	11.7	73.5
SD	4.4	4.1	5.0	4.2	4.1	3.9	19.4

The comparison shows that the mean total score and five of the six mean subscale scores are higher for the neonatal nurses in this study than a group made up of urban hospital nurses from a number of different departments. The range of scores was also wider. Total scores on the NSI were found to be significantly related to a wide range of other variables. A higher total score was found to be associated with: working full-time ($p=<0.001$), rotating shifts ($p=<0.001$), being qualified in specialty ($p=<0.01$), being older ($p=<0.01$), having no children ($p=<0.05$), and being employed in the middle to higher grades ($p=<0.001$). In all types of unit working more, often at unsocial hours, and having more responsibility seem to be what characterises those experiencing most stress in the environment of the neonatal unit.

The profiles of subscale scores for each type of unit were examined. The scores for stress experienced in managing the workload (MW1 and MW2) and dealing with patients and relatives (DPR) were significantly different, with those for regional centres being highest. These and other associations are shown in Table 8.7. with the associated significance levels. In some instances the relationships were not linear. For example, on the first three subscales covering workload and organisational aspects, the highest grades were most affected, though for the other three subscales that have more to do with individual perception of performance in the nursing role, it was the middle grades that experienced more stress. Of the different shifts worked, nurses

Table 8.7 · Significant associations between scores on the subscales of the Nurse Stress Index and aspects of work in neonatal care

Sub-scale	Aspects of neonatal work					
	Unit Type	Grade	Full/Part Time	Shift	QIS	Age
Managing the workload 1.	***	***	***	***	***	
Managing the workload 2.	**	***	***	***	***	
Organisational Support and Involvement		***		*	***	**
Dealing with patients and relatives	*	***	***	***	**	***
Home work conflict		***	**			***
Confidence and competence in role		***			***	

(Mann-Witney U test/Kruskal Wallis * $p=<0.05$ ** $p=<0.01$, *** $p=<0.001$)

employed to rotate between days and nights reported most stress, followed by nurses working days and least was reported by those working nights only. Having children was associated with lower scores on four of the scales, but not surprisingly, those with children experienced more stress in relation to home – work conflict (see Chapter 7).

In the area of health and psychological wellbeing a number of factors are likely to be linked. Obviously the fact that some nurses have children and others do not, is likely to be associated with other characteristics, such as the shift and hours currently worked. Similarly, age is likely to be linked with years of experience and being qualified in specialty. Some of the possible health effects of the stress experienced while working in this area have already been discussed. Using the total score for the NSI, it was found that a higher score was significantly associated with lowered job satisfaction (Pearson's $r=.36$ $p=<0.001$), more illnesses in the last year ($r=.31$, $p=<0.001$) and poorer health currently ($p=<0.001$). That there are these associations and a positive correlation between the NSI and the GHQ12 scores (Pearson's $r=.41$, $p=<0.001$) indicate that there seem to be at least some links between occupational stress and psychological symptoms experienced by nurses working in the environment of neonatal care.

Multivariate Analyses

In order to investigate which explanatory variables best explained the outcome variables being considered (for example NSI score, GHQ score, days off sick, numbers of illnesses) multiple regression analyses were carried out. Outcome variables were deemed to be binomially distributed and a logit link was used. A forward stepwise regression model was employed and explanatory variables were added in according to the magnitude of the decrease in the scaled deviance (minus two times the log likelihood ratio). Variables were added sequentially into the model until the change in deviance was not statistically significant. These analyses were performed using the GENSTAT5 statistical programme. This model did not take any possible "random effects" into consideration.

Once the statistically significant variables had been obtained by stepwise regression, these variables were then read into the statistical package EGRET (SERC, 1985) which also modelled random effects. This was done using the study units as the grouping factor for random effects. Any changes in the size of regression coefficients, their standard errors and statistical significance were noted. The critical significance probability was taken to be 0.05 on a 2-sided null hypothesis of no difference.

The main question that we wished to answer in this area concerned the factors associated with poorer physical and mental health among the neonatal nursing workforce. It was not methodologically possible to link work environment characteristics with individual nurse data as these would have been duplicated for all the nurses in a particular unit. A different study design and a substantial random sample of individuals from a larger number of units, together with detailed information on workload and organisation would be required to address this question fully.

The multiple regression analyses revealed the links summarised in Table 8.8. A reduced set of associated variables resulting from the EGRET analysis is listed in Table 8.9. The robustness of the relationships found are demonstrated by their continued appearance here.

The directions of the relationships found in the EGRET analysis are shown in Table 8.10. From this and the previous tables it is evident that the number of

Table 8.8 · Significant relationships between individual and other factors associated with physical health, psychological wellbeing, occupational stress and perceptions of issues at work found using GENSTAT

Outcome Variables	Associated factors
Physical health	
General health	Life events*** Education***
Number of illnesses	Life events*** Years neonatal nursing*
Days off sick	Life events** Age*
Over/underweight	Partner*
Alcohol consumption	Grade*** Education***
Caffeine consumption	Age***
Smoking	Education***
Psychological wellbeing	
GHQ score	Life events*** Type A/Type B**
Anxiety	Life events* Children***
Depression	Life events*** Partner*** Years neonatal nursing**
Stress and satisfaction	
Job Satisfaction	Children**
Nurse Stress Index	Type A/Type B**
Subscales:	
Managing Workload 1.	Shift*** Grade*** Life Events*
Managing Workload 2.	Grade***
Organisational Support	Age*
Patients and Relatives	Shift*** Grade*
Home–Work Conflict	Grade** Type A/Type B** Dependent children***
Confidence/Competence	QIS*** Age* Type A/Type B*
Perception of work	
Worries about babies	Grade** Type A/Type B**
Worries about unit	Grade*** Type A/Type B*
Worries about staff	Grade*** Type A/Type B* Life events** Children* Family locally* Years neonatal nursing*

* p=<0.05, ** p=<0.01, *** p=<0.001

Table 8.9 · Significant relationships between individual and other factors associated with physical health, psychological wellbeing, occupational stress and perceptions of issues at work found using EGRET

Outcome Variables	Associated factors
Physical health	
General health	Life events***
Number of illnesses	Life events*** Type of unit*
Days off sick	Life events**
Over/underweight	Partner*
Alcohol consumption	
Caffeine consumption	
Smoking	Education***
Psychological wellbeing	
GHQ score	Life events*** Type of unit*
Anxiety	Life events*** Children***
Depression	Life events*** Partner***
Stress and satisfaction	
Job Satisfaction	Children***
Nurse Stress Index Subscales:	
Managing Workload 1.	Shift*** Years Neonatal Nursing** Life Events*
Managing Workload 2.	Grade**
Organisational Support	Age***
Patients and Relatives	
Home–Work Conflict	Dependent children***
Confidence/Competence	QIS*** Age*
Perception of work	
Worries about babies	Grade**
Worries about unit	Grade*
Worries about staff	Grade** Life events**

* p=<0.05, ** p=<0.01, *** p=<0.001

life events experienced by individual nurses in the previous year is the most salient factor. Events that were included among these were the death or illness of a close friend or family member, assault or robbery, separating from a partner and moving house. It is not surprising that when those working in a stressful specialty like neonatal care experience problems outside the working environment, there is also an effect on the way they feel about their work. The protective benefits of having a partner and children are confirmed, though

Table 8.10 · Summary of the direction of the relationships found among the factors included in the EGRET analysis

Variables	Outcomes
More Life Events	Poorer general health More illnesses More days off sick Higher GHQ score More likely to suffer anxiety More likely to be depressed More pressure from workload More worries about inter-staff problems
No Partner	More over/underweight More likely to be depressed
With Children	Less likely to suffer anxiety Higher job satisfaction More home–work conflict
Less Education	More smoking
More years in neonatal nursing	More pressure from workload
Increasing Age	Fewer problems with organisational support
Type of Unit	More illnesses in subregional units Higher GHQ scores in subregional units
Shift	More workload pressure on days only
Grade	Higher grades experience more workload pressure More concerns about babies for higher grades More concerns about unit organisation for higher grades More concerns about staff problems for higher grades
QIS	Less concern about confidence and competence in role

there may be some pressure from the competing demands of work and home. Social support in a wider context was also included as a variable but not found to be significant. Part-time and full-time working was removed from the variables included as there was a close match with those with and without children. Nurses who have worked for longer in neonatal care experience more stress in relation to managing the workload and those in the higher grades, presumably with more responsibility, experience more pressure and worries concerning all aspects of their work in neonatal care.

In summary it seems that the upheaval and distress associated with personal events outside the workplace and the duration and intensity of exposure to the neonatal unit environment both have effects on the health and wellbeing of nurses working in neonatal care.

Stressful Incidents

The Nurse Stress Index can indicate the general problem areas for a particular group of nurses, but neonatal care is a specialty, with its own skills, concerns and unique problems. In order to address the question of what concerns neonatal nurses about their situation and the work that they do, a number of approaches were adopted. Individual nurses were asked to describe a stressful incident or situation that had occurred in the last few months. The reports returned covered a wide range of topics, the most common of which are listed in Table 8.11. The same topics were most often referred to by staff working in the different kinds of unit, though the rankings varied. Overall the most frequent topic was unit organisation, management and staffing arrangements. This was followed by sick babies, dealing with parents, nurse–nurse communication, workload, death and nurse training and experience.

Many incidents combined a variety of elements:

> 'We were short of staff, with poor medical cover and yet we had to ventilate a premature baby who was critically ill. Medical staff were not qualified and experienced enough to manage the case, but unable to transfer the baby to another unit. The parents were extremely angry with our unit which they labelled as inadequate and

Table 8.11 · Topics referred to by nurses in reporting on stressful incidents in the different types of unit (n=24 units)

			Stressful incident topics	
Regional units				
	Rank	1	Unit organisation	35%
		2	Parents	20%
		3	Sick babies	19%
		4	Nurse training and experience	18%
		5	Workload	16%
			Nurse–nurse communication	16%
Subregional units				
	Rank	1	Sick babies	30%
		2	Parents	20%
		3	Death	20%
		4	Nurse–nurse communication	18%
		5	Unit organisation	17%
District units				
	Rank	1	Unit organisation	32%
		2	Sick babies	25%
		3	Workload	21%
		4	Nurse–nurse communication	20%
		5	Unit management	19%

useless. Trying to cope with the emergency, and at the same time to gain trust and understanding with the parents was very stressful.'

'A term baby died at four weeks of age. There was very little time to deal with the parents adequately on my shift, but I made sure that they and their baby had one nurse to look after them on the night shift. The baby died at midnight. Next day the parents arrived at midday and were shown to the quiet room where they had been with their baby. The equipment and other things had not even been cleared away!'

'I was working in a low dependency area as a fairly new student member of staff and allocated to a cubicle with five babies I had never nursed before. Most of the equipment was new to me, the report was brief as the nurse was already late for her half day. I was working on my own, trying to figure out alien fluid charts for the babies who all had a combination of IV and oral feeds and answer various enquiries from parents who had come to visit. On top of that I was told that I was expecting a new admission, having never even witnessed the admission procedure for this hospital, let alone done one.'

Others relate to a specific problem area such as workload:

'Last week on a shift I was the only trained member of staff in the intensive room. Caring for three intensive care babies, who were quite unstable at times and needing a lot of care (IVI's, IAI's and naso-gastric feeding, IV antibiotics and other medication). I was rushed all shift and felt upset I couldn't give each baby the care and full attention they needed. The nurse in charge was too busy to help me.'

or staffing:

'I was in charge of the unit and we were closed to admissions as we were very busy and short staffed. I was on night duty. A mother was admitted to delivery suite in early labour with 31 week twins. I was put under a great deal of pressure to take the babies and in the end I had to telephone the unit leader at home at 1am as I felt I could not take them without more staff. She got out of bed and came to work herself, to look after the babies.'

'Recently we had to refuse to take a child for ventilation because we had no staff to look after it, even though we knew that the adult ICU was full. At the time I had already spent a lot of time finding staff to look after the babies we already had in the unit.'

'I was on a shift with three staff on (one a nursery nurse), to 8 babies, 3 being ventilated, and expected to look after these babies on my own, as well as be on call for labour suite. The nursing officer believed we'd cope, since we had used up our monthly budget for agency nurses.'

Incidents concerning nurse–nurse communication took different forms, but more often a less senior member of staff reported the incident and a relatively senior member of staff was the subject:

'I came on duty for a late shift and found a member of staff from the early shift in tears and totally demoralised following an incident earlier when the senior sister had shouted and lectured her in front of parents, medical staff, and other colleagues.'

'When I rang in sick, as I had been signed off work for a week by a medical certificate, I was told by the senior nurse on the unit that she did not believe I was ill and that I only wanted a few extra days off and only came to work when I felt like it. I felt bad enough being off sick and the attitude of the person in charge did nothing but add to the stress.'

Slightly less frequently mentioned (10% of incidents) was nurse–doctor conflict:

'There was a difference of opinion between myself (experienced sister in charge) and a fairly new SHO, on the best treatment for a baby. On the ward round later it turned out that my treatment would have been correct after all. I find it difficult to work with SHOs who have the attitude that "I'm the doctor, you're just the nurse", especially when we have had to instruct and supervise them doing technical procedures'.

'A 26 week baby was transferred back from an ICU at another hospital at 48 hours of age and began to have recurrent apnoea attacks. The consultant was informed and told the inexperienced SHO to arrange transfer back to the other hospital, but he did not visit. The SHO had to go to labour ward for LSCS, leaving me with sole care of the baby whilst waiting for the paediatric team to arrive.'

Stressful incidents and situations while dealing with sick babies and their parents are a regular feature of work in the neonatal unit:

'The death of a baby, coping with bereavement of parents I had only just met. Difficulty in performing last offices on the child as I was also responsible for another ventilated baby who was also quite unstable. Lack of support due to a shortage of staff. My dilemma was that I knew they needed me to stay with them and support them, but I was needed for intensive care work on the unit.'

'Having to deal with the admission of a baby with non-accidental injury, accompanying the mother and boyfriend to see the paediatrician. I had to physically walk ahead of this couple to prevent me reacting badly towards them.'

'When I had done my best and some parents still thought their baby was not being looked after "properly" and said so, questioning my professional judgement.'

Experience and training, though they may facilitate coping with abnormalities and death, do not render nurses insensitive to what is their key task of caring:

'A ventilated baby was transferred back to my unit with an inoperable heart condition. We and the parents had been told that the baby would die soon after being extubated. He lived for three weeks. As someone involved in his care I found this very stressful.'

'A terminally ill baby was dying very slowly. Her condition was very poor and quality of life was very poor. I found it upsetting nursing her because I knew I would not wish my baby to die in hospital in such a way and felt it would be better for her to die quickly rather than taking months to slowly deteriorate'.

'A new baby was born with a major heart defect and was rejected by her parents, who didn't want any treatment for her. I held the baby until she died two hours later.'

A wide range of topics in addition to those mentioned were also described. These included equipment problems and shortages, training, mistakes, grading, safety and problems with other departments. The incidents detailed by individual nurses and the issues raised show that these are not peculiar to just one or two work situations or to the individual nurses concerned. In both describing stressful incidents and suggesting changes to alleviate stress in their unit (Table 8.12.), there is a considerable degree of consensus in the profession as a whole about the most salient issues.

Table 8.12 · Areas where nurses perceive that improvement and change is needed to alleviate stress in the working environment of neonatal care

			Improvements suggested	
Regional units				
	Rank	1	Staffing	54%
		2	Working relationships	16%
		3	Unit organisation	12%
Subregional units				
	Rank	1	Staffing	31%
		2	Working relationships	29%
		3	Unit organisation	11%
			Teaching and training	11%
District units				
	Rank	1	Staffing	46%
		2	Working relationships	21%
		3	Unit organisation	11%

Nurses' Perceptions of the Neonatal Unit

Not all stress is experienced by the nursing staff as distress, and many spoke positively about working in neonatal care:

> 'I enjoy this specialty, we are lucky to be working in neonatal medicine.'

> 'Neonatal nursing is demanding but very rewarding.'

> 'I really enjoy working in the neonatal environment with all the stresses and strains it brings with it.'

For some, working under pressure and doing a good job is very satisfying:

> 'I find neonatal nursing stimulating, fulfilling and continually changing, providing a constant challenge to adapt appropriately. I would recommend this field of work to those looking for a challenging, rewarding career.'

As a way of collecting comparable data from all the nurses in the study, adjective checklists were used in several different contexts. Mixed, but equal numbers of positive and negative terms were presented. Those most frequently selected are shown in Tables 8.13. and 8.14.

Table 8.13 · The adjectives most frequently used to describe the unit "as a place to work" (n=718 nurses)

		Adjectives used	
		Positive	**Negative**
Rank	1	Challenging	Frustrating
	2	Rewarding	Pressurised
	3	Satisfying	Annoying
	4	Stimulating	Authoritarian
	5	Fulfilling	Stagnating

The terms selected reflect the often mixed and ambivalent feelings that neonatal nurses have about the neonatal unit as a workplace. They also confirm the views expressed more graphically in the individual stressful incident descriptions and other comments about their job. Not only are some nurses concerned about how they view their unit, they are aware of how others might see them, especially newcomers:

> 'The general atmosphere on the unit is friendly and relaxed, it is hard work and sometimes to the uninitiated seems very confusing and unorganised. Although I have been on the unit for some years and am a fairly confident person I am concerned by the perceptions new and inexperienced staff come away with. We are a friendly

Table 8.14 · The adjectives most frequently used to describe "the atmosphere in the unit" (n=718 nurses)

		Adjectives used	
		Positive	**Negative**
Rank	1	Friendly	Hectic
	2	Cheerful	Cliquey
	3	Efficient	Tense
	4	Organised	Chaotic
	5	Welcoming	Disorganised

bunch but when busy and overstretched I feel that we do not give them the support and encouragement they need.'

In fact a third of nurses said they felt unsupported at work and some felt that the answer was to move to another unit or area of nursing. At the time of the study more than a third (36%) of those working in neonatal care were thinking of finding another job in nursing. Some (34%) even had thoughts about leaving the profession and finding an occupation other than nursing.

Issues and Concerns in Neonatal Nursing

The nurses were also asked about the issues and concerns that worried them while working in their unit. Table 8.15. shows the proportion that were concerned in the area of caring for babies.

Infant pain and suffering experienced in the course of neonatal care was found to be a major concern, as was infant death after prolonged treatment.

Table 8.15 · Proportion of nurses expressing concern about different aspects of their work in caring for babies in neonatal units (n=718)

Caring for babies	
Infant pain and suffering	85%
Long term outcome	77%
Infant death after prolonged treatment	63%
Questionable attempts at resuscitation	60%
Babies < 24 weeks gestation	56%
Nursing a baby with abnormalities incompatible with life	53%
Making a mistake while caring for a baby	52%
Caring for a terminally ill baby	47%

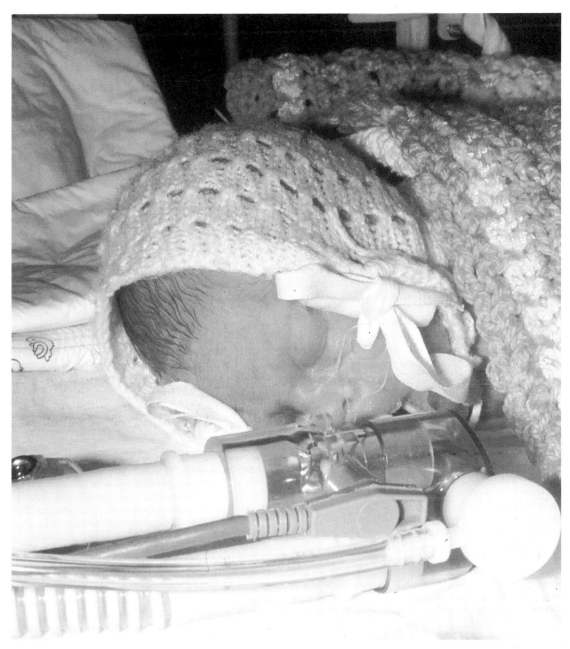

A sick preterm baby requiring ventilation

Table 8.16 · The proportions of nurses expressing concern about different aspects of neonatal unit organisation (n=718 nurses)

Unit organisation

Having to cut corners in order to get work done	75%
Shortage of skilled nursing staff	75%
Feeling pressured to accept babies when unit full	63%
Working with staff of unknown ability	63%
Nursing responsibility for new medical staff	53%

The possibility of litigation seems to be becoming an important issue for many nurses and more than half of those in the study indicated this was a concern to them. Even after a shift is finished many nurses worry about having done the right thing, filled in the right forms and having written up the notes fully.

Concerns in the area of unit organisation predominantly revolved around workload, staff shortages and the need for skilled staff Table 8.16. Responsibility for new medical staff, heightened at change-over times, also worried a large proportion of nurses. A lack of a clear cut policies in many areas is also felt to be a concern and a contributor to stress by nearly half the nurses in the study.

Nurses were less concerned about inter-staff relationships than about caring for sick babies or the organisational problems of neonatal care. However, all the issues listed in Table 8.17. were of concern to nearly a quarter or more of those working in neonatal care. In the enclosed and relatively isolated environment of the neonatal unit poor communication and interpersonal problems can markedly affect the quality of the working environment, both for those directly involved and those less so. Unit morale and personal motivation can be affected by particular individuals and long-established modes of working:

Table 8.17 · The proportions of nurses expressing concern about different aspects of inter-staff relationships in the context of neonatal care (n=718 nurses)

Inter-staff relationships and problems

One-way communication	36%
Conflict of nursing and management goals	30%
Personality problems	25%
Effects of "burn-out"	23%
Nurse–nurse conflict	22%

'Although I enjoy my work very much and I have an open mind, stress levels depend upon who one is working with on any particular shift.'

'The only changes allowed on the unit are consultant orientated – We're not allowed to make suggestions. Routines are strict. On night duty the decisions have to wait for the day staff. It is very frustrating. I only work on the unit when forced.'

'The manager of the unit comes to work as she gets up, is uncaring towards her staff's feelings and has a bad communication problem. The atmosphere when she is in charge is stifling and whatever you do is wrong'.

Sometimes the problems are more general:

'Working on SCBU and enjoying the job depends a lot on inter-personal relationships. In some instances senior staff are extremely helpful and encouraging. Unfortunately this motivating atmosphere is not constant.'

'Neonatal nursing is very stressful and good teamwork is needed, unfortunately, where I work, different grades of nurses work well in their own grade, but not as a whole team, I feel this is because of the big age gap between us and the senior sisters, who I am sure see younger nurses as a threat.'

Inter-Unit Differences

In the course of the study it became clear that there were differences between neonatal units in their organisation and management and also in respect of the wellbeing and morale of the staff working in them. The factors that may be contributing to low or high sickness rates, anxiety, depression and low job satisfaction are difficult to track down and quantify. Though it is possible that each unhappy unit may be unhappy in its own way, several attempts were made to tease out possible links.

In looking to account for factors associated with wellbeing and links with staffing and unit variables a principal components analysis (with varimax rotation) was carried out using SPSS/PC+4. This type of analysis was carried out in order to determine which combination of the selected variables accounted for the maximum variance; the remaining variance accounted for by the next independent combination of the same variables and so on. The organisational variables entered were the size of the nursing establishment, total cots, intensive care cots, admissions, the proportion of F–I grade staff and the proportion qualified in specialty. The unit wellbeing variables were mean NSI, GHQ and satisfaction scores, mean days off sick, and proportions of staff unwell, depressed, smoking and markedly over or underweight.

The principal component, accounting for 35% of the variance was associated with size and type of unit and all the organisational variables were grouped here. The following components were each largely dependent on a single variable: the GHQ variable accounting for 18%, the job satisfaction variable for 11%, the current health variable for 9% and sick leave and smoking for 6 and 5% respectively. It seems that the size and to some extent the type of unit were the dominating influence overwhelming the other variables.

In another approach the 24 units' average days sick leave and illnesses per nurse, mean scores on the GHQ12, the NSI, and job satisfaction, and the proportion of staff suffering from anxiety and depression, were examined in relation to the degree of under or overstaffing in those units (see model 2 in Chapter 3). No significant correlations were found, probably due to the large inter-unit variation, though two concerned with managing the workload and the average number of days taken as sick leave did approach significance (Pearson's $r=.37$, $p=<0.08$; $r=.39$, $p=<0.057$).

The unit average scores on the GHQ, NSI, job satisfaction, days sick leave, and illness totals and the proportion of the staff suffering from anxiety and depression were also used to produce a measure of unit wellbeing. Each score or proportion was ranked and a combined rank produced. The rankings were then examined in relation to variables that included the size of the unit and the proportion of staff qualified in specialty. Again, probably due to the inter-unit differences discussed in Chapters 3 and 4 and the small subject numbers (24 units), few significant relationships were found. "Unhappy" units included regional centres, subregional and district units and though pressure from workload and organisational difficulties were evident, these varied in nature and were not the only notable features in the working environment of these units. There was a significant relationship ($p=<0.001$) between the combined ranking on unit wellbeing and a rating made on senior nursing and medical support and leadership. Having supportive, approachable and motivated management and leadership marked out the more fortunate units, in contrast to those ranked lowest where, without support, the dominant theme was one of apathy and helplessness.

Caring for the Carers

Nurses are members of a profession in which they have responsibility for people rather than things. With small sick babies as their patients this responsibility is magnified for neonatal nurses. The imbalance between the demands of the job and the ability to meet these demands is not simply a reflection of the individuals working in this specialty. In their working environment these nurses are commonly expected to control their feelings, minimise attachment, utilise their skills and behave professionally. Detachment and denial of feelings, ritual task performance, making checks and counter-checks, formal distribution of responsibility, reprimand and the avoidance of change are among the strategies used to deal with emotional stress (Menzies, 1970).

In the environment of the neonatal unit such tactics may have short-term validity, but are unlikely to succeed in the longer term as they do not address the most salient issues, from either the point of view of the individual or the organisation. It seems that neonatal nurses are stressed. The nature of the work they have to carry out, that is factors intrinsic to neonatal nursing, obviously contribute. However, it seems that many in neonatal nursing accept the unique forms of stress they are subject to as part of their professional role but may be reacting with dissatisfaction and alienation to administrative stressors which they regard as avoidable. The comments that some nurses made as they filled out the questionnaires showed that they were clearly quite concerned and distressed about how they were feeling and about the way that colleagues were behaving at times. Further development of support and counselling services, at present available in a few units, would undoubtedly help some individuals. Conventionally those working in the caring professions have been expected to put their personal problems on one side when coming to work. However, many it seems are unable to do so and they and their attitudes to work are affected by them. The strong links between important life events and sickness and wellbeing indicate that more management awareness in this area is needed. Practical steps include increased compassionate and carer's leave where necessary, a flexible attitude to temporary alterations in hours and "stress days" taken by individual nurses as necessary. Most units did not report having initiatives designed to improve staff support, neither did they facilitate variable working patterns nor show imaginative use of leave arrangements. Frequent monitoring and audit of sickness data and schemes which include non-judgemental interviews following return after sickness absence are essential in the best interests of both staff and management (Seccombe and Buchan, 1993). Greater use of occupational health screening prior to and in the course of employment, as recently recommended (Clothier, 1994) is essential. More generally, agreed and written unit policies, improved orientation programmes for nursing and junior medical staff, increased educational opportunities for staff at different levels to refresh skills and extend competence, support mechanisms with both formal and informal elements and acknowledgement of staffing problems when they arise can all be part of the process by which neonatal care itself can be appraised and developed.

Support and awareness of the problems of individual nurses may assist in improving the situation. However, the work stresses experienced as a function of staffing and related problems in the working environment of the neonatal unit itself, are unlikely to alter substantially unless the issues discussed in Chapters 3, 4,and 5 are also addressed. As in the areas of staffing, skill mix and training, inter-unit differences were also found here. That the proportion of staff suffering from anxiety in different units ranged from none to more than a third in the units studied and that sickness rates in some units were more than three times those found elsewhere must be of interest to those managing and those purchasing services.

While neonatal nurses work in an intrinsically stressful environment and many are experiencing the effects of stress, there are also rewards intrinsic to giving this kind of nursing care. Seeing the changes and improvements that are the result of their skilled professional care and babies going home with their own families is a vital part of the positive side of the work equation.

References

Audit Commission (1994) Trusting in the Future: Towards an Audit Agenda for NHS Providers. HMSO, London.

Astbury, J. and Yu, V. H. Y. (1982). Determinants of stress for staff in a neonatal intensive care unit. *Arch. Dis. Childhood*, **57**, 108.

Barton, J., Spelton, E. R., Smith, I., Totterdell, P. A. and Folkard, S. (1993a) Night and shift work in nursing and midwifery. Unpublished report to the Department of Health.

Barton, J., Spelton, E. R., Smith, I., Totterdell, P. A. and Folkard, S. (1993b) A classification of nursing and midwifery shift systems. *Int. J. Nursing Studies*, **30**, 65–80.

Bellig, L. (1980). The expanded nursing role in the neonatal intensive care unit. *Clinics in Perinatology*, 7, 159–171.

Bender, H. (1981). Experiences in running a nursing staff group in a hospital intensive care unit. *J.Child Psychotherapy*, 7, 20–28.

Blaxter, M. (1990). Health and Lifestyles. Routledge, London.

Bohle, P. and Tilley, A. J. (1989) The impact of nightwork on psychological wellbeing. *Ergonomics* **32**, 9, 1089–1099.

Bortner, R. W. and Rosenman, R. H. (1967) The measurement of Pattern A behaviour. *J. Chron. Dis.*, **20**: 525–533.

Bowling, A. (1991) Measuring Health. OUP, Milton Keynes.

Brown, D., Carson, J., Fagin, L., Bartlett, H. and Leary, J. (1994) Coping with caring. *Nursing Times*, **90**, 53–55.

Clothier, C. (1994) The Allit Inquiry – Independent inquiry relating to the deaths and injuries on the childrens' ward at Grantham and Kesteven General Hospital during the period Feb–Apr 1991. HMSO, London.

Coffey, L., Skipper, J. and Jung, F. (1988) Nurses and shift work: effects on job performance and job-related stress. *Journal of Advanced Nursing*, **13**, 245–254.

Consolvo C. A.(1979). Nurse turnover in the newborn intensive care unit. *JOGN Nursing*, July/Aug, 201–204.

Cooper, C. L. and Marshall, J. (1976) Occupational sources of stress: a review of the literature relating to coronary heart disease and mental ill health. *J. Occup. Psychol.*, **49**: 11–28.

Cooper, C. L. and Payne, R. (1978) Stress at Work, Chichester, Wiley.

Cooper, P., Campbell, E., Day, A., Kennerley, H. and Bond, A. (1988) Psychiatric disorder after childbirth: a prospective study of prevalence, incidence, course and nature. *British Journal of Psychiatry*, **152**, 799–806.

Dewe, P. J. (1987) Identifying strategies nurses use to cope with work stress. *Journal of Advanced Nursing*, **12**, 489–497.

Davidson, M. J. and Cooper, C. L. (1980) Type A coronary-prone behaviour and stress in senior female managers and administrators. *J. Occup. Med.*, **22**: 801–805.

Davidson, M. J. and Cooper, C. L. (1983) Stress and the Woman Manager. Oxford: Robertson.

Duxbury, M. (1984). Head nurse leadership style with staff burn-out and job satisfaction in neonatal intensive care units. *Nursing Research*, **33**, 97–101.

Goldberg, D. (1978) Manual of the General Health Questionnaire. NFER, Windsor.

Goldberg, D. and Williams, P. (1988). A User's Guide to the General Health Questionnaire. NFER-Nelson, Windsor, Berks.

Gray-Toft, P. and Anderson, J. G.(1981). Stress among hospital nursing staff: its causes and effects. *Social Science Medicine*, **15a**, 639–647.

Harris, P., Hingley, P. and Cooper, C. (1988) Nurse Stress Index. Resource Assessment and Development, Harrogate.

Hingley, P. and Cooper, C.(1986) Stress and the Nurse Manager. Wiley, Chichester.

Jacobson, S. F. (1978). Stressful situations for neonatal intensive care nurses. *American Journal of Maternal-Child Nursing*, **3**, 144–150.

Jacobson, S. F. (1983). Stresses and coping strategies of neonatal intensive care nurses. *Research in Nursing and Health*, **6**, 33–40.

Kumar, R. and Robson, K. (1984) A prospective study of emotional disorders in childbearing women. *British Journal of Psychiatry*, **144**, 35–47.

Lachman, V. D. (1983) Stress Management. Grune and Stratton, New York.

Lazarus, R. S. (1976) Patterns of Adjustment. McGraw Hill, New York.

Marshall, R. E. and Kasman C. (1980). Burn-out in the neonatal intensive care unit. *Paediatrics*, **65**, 1161–1165.

Metropolitan Life (1983)

Menzies, I. E. P. (1970) The Functioning of Social Systems as a Defence Against Anxiety: A Report on a Study of the Nursing Service of a General Hospital. The Tavistock Institute of Human Relations, London.

O'Hara, M., Neunaber, D. and Zekoski, E. (1986) A prospective study of postpartum depression: prevalence, course and predictive factors. *Journal of Abnormal Psychology*, **93**, 158–171.

Parkes, K. R. (1985). Stressful episodes reported by first-year student nurses. *Social Science Medicine*, **20**, 945–953.

Payne, R. and Firth-Cozens, J. (1987) Stress in Health Professionals. Wiley, Chichester.

Spelton, E. R., Smith, Totterdell, P. A. I., Barton, J., Folkard, S. and Bohle, P. (1993) The relationship between coping strategies and GHQ scores in nurses. *Ergonomics* **36**, 227–232.

Seccombe, I. and Ball, J, (1992) Motivation, Morale and Mobility: A Profile of Qualified Nurses in the 1990's. IMS Report No 233. IMS Brighton.

Seccomb, I. and Buchan, J. (1993) Absent Nurses: The Costs and Consequences. IMS Report No 259, IMS, Brighton.

SERC (1985) EGRET, SERC, Seattle, USA.

Strickland, M., Spector, S., Hamelin-Cook, P., Hanna, C., Moore, C., Bellig, L. and Fiorato A. (1980). Nurse training and staffing in the neonatal intensive care unit. *Clinics in Perinatology*, 7, 173–186.

Tyler, P. A. and Ellison, R. N. (1994) Sources of stress and psychological wellbeing in high dependency nursing. *Journal of Advanced Nursing*, **19**, 469–476.

Waldron, I. (1978) Type A behaviour pattern and coronary heart disease in men and women. *Soc. Sci. Med.*, **12**b:167–170.

Walker, C. (1982), Neonatal intensive care and stress. *Archives of Disease in Childhood*, **57**, 85–88.

Watson, J., Elliott, S., Rugg, A. and Brough, D. (1984) Psychiatric disorder in pregnancy and the first postnatal year. *British Journal of Psychiatry*, **144**, 453–462.

Chapter 9 · Parents and Neonatal Care

Parents' Experience of Neonatal Care

The birth and subsequent admission of an infant for specialised neonatal care is a time of upheaval and stress for parents (Klaus and Kennell, 1982; Redshaw, Rivers and Rosenblatt, 1985). The impact of the hospital neonatal unit environment and circumstances surrounding the birth or unexpected admission are thought to have a powerful influence on the psychological and social adjustment of parents to their role and to the parent-infant relationship (Jeffcoate et al, 1979; Greene et al, 1983; de Chateau and Wiberg, 1984).

For a family, having a baby in neonatal care often presents as a psycho-social crisis. Parents with a newborn, critically ill or high-risk infant have anxieties about what is currently happening, concerns about the future and their own ability to parent such a child, both at the time and as he or she develops. The environment is usually strange and unfamiliar; it is often noisy and crowded with technical equipment; there are large numbers of medical and nursing staff working as multiple caretakers and givers of information and establishing satisfactory communication can be difficult. Parents are also confronted with the reactions and feelings of relatives and friends (McHaffie, 1989; 1990).

Thus the way in which parents experience neonatal care is dependent on many factors. The nursing and medical staff, by what they do and say, can affect how parents feel at the time and subsequently. The way a unit is run and organised, the policies and how they are put into practice, are all elements that contribute to parents' sense of wellbeing, confidence and trust. Unanswered questions and fear about expressing anxieties and negative feelings can affect parenting in a normal context, but where babies are sick and mothers and fathers separated from them, the problems may be compounded.

This part of the present study aimed to document and explore some of the issues for a large number of families whose babies had been in-patients in a wide range of hospital neonatal units. Focusing on the needs and perceptions of parents at this critical time, the study was less oriented towards their psychological responses and longer term adjustment and more towards aspects of the organisation and management of neonatal care that may be amenable to intervention and improvement. Parents as consumers of this part of the health care system were thus the focus here.

A large number of parents whose babies had been recently cared for in 23 of the 24 study units (see Chapter 2 for details of recruitment) were contacted and sent questionnaires two months after the baby's discharge home. They were

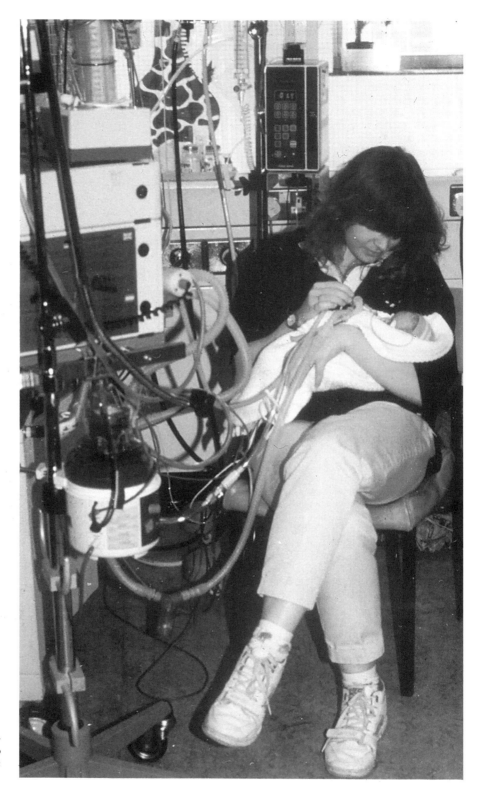

A mother enjoys a brief cuddle with her very small baby who is being ventilated in intensive care

thus a totally unselected group of babies and families. The high return rate of 80% reflects on the motivation and interest of this group of parents whose newborn babies had required neonatal care. The topics covered by the questionnaire included aspects of the pregnancy, birth, reactions to the admission of their baby to a neonatal unit, involvement in care, perceptions of the NNU and use of the facilities provided. A mixture of structured and open-ended questions, including adjective checklists, was used.

Who goes to neonatal care?

The characteristics of the full sample of 456 babies on whom questionnaires were returned were as follows: 55% were male and 45% were female; 86% were from singleton births, 14% from twin births and one from a larger multiple birth. The births took place in 54 different hospitals in England and the reasons for admission to neonatal care are presented by unit type and overall in Table 9.1.

The gestational age and birthweight distributions for the sample (including those of the babies who died) are shown in Figures 9.1 and 9.2. From these and the table it can be seen that many of the babies admitted to the study units were preterm, of low birth weight, had breathing difficulties and a wide range of other problems including suspected abnormalities. As might be expected, preterm birth is the major factor in admission to neonatal care and examination of the gestational age data shows that more than two-thirds (69%) of the study infants were born at less than 37 weeks completed gestation and 31% were born at less than 33 weeks gestational age.

The distribution of mothers by age group was as follows: 8% were under 20 years of age; 65% between 20 and 30 years of age; 27% between 31 and 40, and 1% were over 40 years of age. Nearly all the mothers (93%) had a partner at this time, more than half of the sample (51%) had other children and 22% had children under two years of age. A large proportion of babies (39%) were delivered by caesarean section, most as an emergency (31%) and some as a planned procedure (8%). A further 9% had operative vaginal deliveries.

The total duration of stay in neonatal care for the study babies ranged from 2–195 days. The distribution (Figure 9.3) shows that the majority (71%) of these babies stayed four weeks or less. However, a small, though significant proportion in terms of their sickness and the care required (12%), stayed for more than twice this time. A very small proportion of babies, not included in the study for the reasons explained in Chapter 2 were transferred to paediatric units for longer term care.

The Introduction to Neonatal Care

The way in which parents are told that their baby's condition will necessitate admission to a neonatal unit and their first experience of the environment can have potent and long-lasting effects. Details of the experience of the 420 study

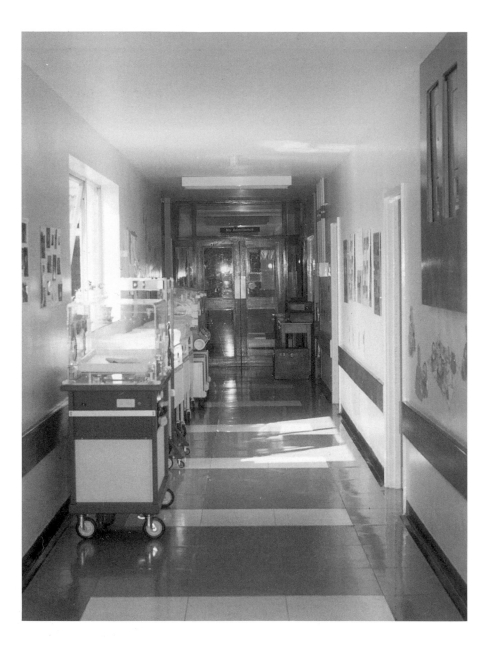

The long corridor leading to the neonatal unit

Table 9.1 · Reasons for admission to neonatal care for study population babies (%)

Reason for Admission	Type of Unit			
	Regional (n=150)	Subregional (n=149)	District (n=157)	All units (n=456)
Prematurity	54.7	52.4	55.6	52.9
Breathing Problems	44.0	38.9	28.0	36.8
Suspected Abnormalities	12.0	2.0	2.9	5.3
Small for Dates	6.0	6.0	6.4	6.1
Birth Trauma	3.3	3.4	3.8	3.5
Cerebral Irritation	1.3	2.0	0.0	1.1
Infection	6.0	3.4	5.7	4.8
Jaundice	2.7	4.0	7.0	4.6
Feeding Problems	3.3	8.0	21.0	11.0
Maternal Problems	4.3	4.9	7.6	5.6
Hypoglycaemia	4.0	8.7	10.8	7.9
Hypothermia	4.0	6.0	5.1	5.0
Haematological Problems	3.3	0.0	2.6	2.0
Observation	7.3	11.4	8.3	9.0

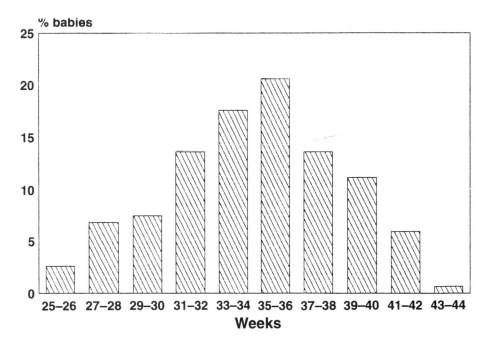

Figure 9.1 · Distribution of study babies by gestational age (n=453 babies)

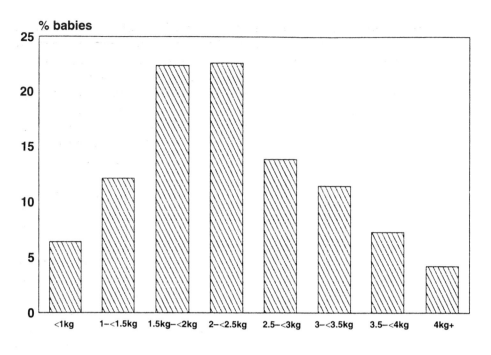

Figure 9.2 · Distribution of study babies by birthweight (n=456)

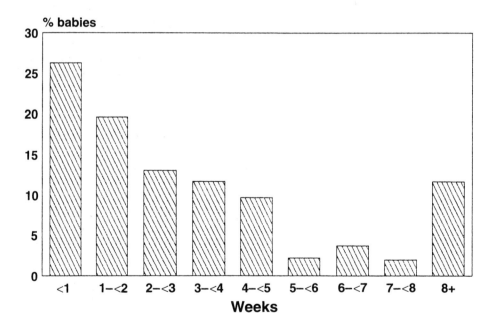

Figure 9.3 · Distribution of study babies by total duration of stay (n=453 babies)

mothers whose babies survived are shown in Table 9.2. (Information about the experiences of the twelve mothers whose babies died are presented separately in the section on bereaved parents. Different questionnaires were used with this group and their data have not been included in the general sections that follow.)

For parents the introduction to neonatal care can occur in a variety of ways. How the pregnancy is experienced and the previous perinatal history create different contexts within which to view and construct what happens in neonatal care. For at-risk mothers, some of whom have been in hospital antenatally, the possibility of their baby needing care in a neonatal unit may have been discussed with them before the birth. A total of 53% of the 420 mothers studied had been admitted to hospital for an antenatal stay at least once during the pregnancy; 19% had more than one stay and 44% had a stay in the month prior to the birth. (The range was from 1–98 days, with a median of 14 days). Mothers who had a previous baby in a neonatal unit (22%) may also have become aware earlier of the need for their current baby to be admitted. For those mothers moved to another hospital shortly before, and during labour, as "in utero transfers" (13%), the circumstances were different yet again.

Similarly, those hearing the neonatal unit mentioned for the first time at the delivery or later, on the post-natal ward, experienced another situation, giving rise to different feelings and attitudes. Knowing earlier may allow time for preparation, but also for continuing anxiety, while hearing later there is no build-up of worries, but instead a sudden realization or shock. The timing of when parents first became aware that their baby would require admission to the neonatal unit is shown for the different gestational age groups (Table 9.3).

Seeing their baby in a neonatal unit is very different from hearing about it and many mothers were not in the best condition to cope with what is for many a frightening and shocking initial experience. A large proportion had experienced high levels of obstetric intervention and 31% had received a general anaesthetic.

Table 9.2 · Maternal experience of care in pregnancy and the perinatal period (n=420 mothers)

% Sample	Unit Type			
	Regional (n=134)	Subregional (n=135)	District (n=151)	All units (n=420)
Previous baby in a neonatal unit	21.6	20.7	22.5	21.7
Antenatal stay	48.1	50.4	58.9	53.0
More than one antenatal stay	23.1	10.4	23.2	19.1
A-N Stay during last month	40.3	38.5	51.7	43.9
Intra-Uterine Transfer	20.2	14.1	6.7	13.3
Infant Transfer Immediately Post-Delivery	26.1	16.3	10.6	17.4

Table 9.3 · When parents first knew their baby would be admitted to neonatal care according to gestational age at birth

% Sample	Gestational Age (weeks)				
	<29 (n=38)	29–32 (n=94)	33–36 (n=174)	>37 (n=138)	All Babies (n=444)
Early pregnancy	13.2	5.3	6.3	8.0	7.2
Later pregnancy	13.2	17.0	11.5	3.7	10.4
In labour	50.0	35.1	23.0	–	20.8
Post-delivery	23.7	37.2	43.7	49.3	42.5
First 24 hours	–	4.3	13.2	26.8	14.5
>24 hours after birth	–	–	2.3	11.6	4.5

This contrasts with the experience of a conventional population of postnatal mothers whose babies do not require admission to a neonatal unit. Indeed, when asked about their health following the birth, 45% of the mothers described themselves as tired and uncomfortable, 8% as exhausted all the time and 12% as very ill. Also contrasting with the "normal" situation, a significant proportion (17%) of these mothers experienced separation from their baby in an immediate way, for their baby's condition had required that he or she be moved to another hospital within a few hours of birth. Only a small number of mothers were able to accompany their baby at this time.

First impressions of the neonatal unit environment can be overwhelming whether you have come from the post-natal ward in the same hospital or from a small unit to a large centre. On first seeing their baby in neonatal care some features of the situation worry and concern parents more than others. Those that were found to concern them most at this stage are listed below in Table 9.4. At this point the baby's appearance and the surrounding equipment are what predominated in terms of importance to parents:

'She was so tiny and there were so many wires"

'He was so small and vulnerable.'

'He looked so still, with all the equipment attached to him'

The baby and his or her immediate environment are what parents mostly focus on at this time. But it is also the point in time when staff begin to explain the baby's condition and tell parents about the unit. Though nursing and medical staff may need to do so, what is said at this time is relatively poorly remembered by most parents (Table 9.5).

For many the admission of their baby to a neonatal unit comes as a complete shock and they are overwhelmed by emotion:

'I felt totally useless. I was so ill and she was so small'

'I was so shocked with it all, not having been to a unit ever before'

'I felt inadequate. I was unable to help my babies and frightened that they might die'

At such a time of stress parents need a great deal of support and reassurance. Some is found in the unit itself, both in terms of the organisation and the large amount of visible equipment, so that they are reassured by seeing their baby settled as comfortably as possible in the difficult circumstances. However, as Table 9.6. shows, for the majority of parents feeling that there were skilled and experienced nurses looking after their baby was what was most important.

Table 9.4 · Aspects of the neonatal care situation that concerned parents when they first saw their baby (n=420)

Aspects of Neonatal Care	% Parents
Equipment	55.6
Baby's appearance	52.7
Noise	38.7
Temperature	27.3
Busy atmosphere	14.0
What doctor said	11.6
What nurse said	10.9

Table 9.5 · Aspects of the neonatal care situation remembered most by parents on first seeing their baby (n=420)

Aspects of Neonatal Care	% Parents
Their baby	78.2
Their own feelings	39.2
The equipment	39.2
The environment	4.3
Other babies	2.9
Medical staff	0.7
Nursing staff	4.3
Previous experience	2.3

Table 9.6 · Aspects of the neonatal care situation that reassured parents most on first seeing their baby (n=420)

Aspects of Neonatal Care	% Parents
The nurses	70.8
Seeing their baby	45.8
The doctors	28.7
The hospital/SCBU	16.6
The equipment	9.9
Other babies	7.0

Handing over responsibility to trained professionals was a common element:

'The nurses seemed so calm and efficient and to know just what they were doing.'

'We were both relieved that she was in the best possible place'

'I knew that although he wasn't with me, he was in safe hands.'

While it is not possible to prepare parents for the crisis that the birth of a preterm or sick baby brings, some familiarity with the neonatal unit environment may help. However, preparation and introduction to the neonatal unit is not part of every hospitals' antenatal course for parents. Among the 24 units on which policy and other data were collected, in only 14 (58%), were groups of parents routinely shown the neonatal unit as part of the preparation for parenthood. In the other hospitals, individual parents were shown round under "special circumstances" and of the study parents only 20% had visited a unit antenatally. Despite doubts expressed by professionals about the value of such visits, they could be seen as part of the information sharing process in which parents can participate. Where it is not possible to show the unit and equipment to parents in advance, the use of audio-visual and photographic material is used in some hospitals and is being received very positively by families, especially when there are problems with maternal illness or visiting arrangements and other children to consider.

What does seem to be encouraging for the staff caring for babies and their families is that most parents have a positive memory of the unit as shown by the adjectives listed in Table 9.7. Overall more positive terms were used than negative terms and the majority of NNUs specialising in this type of care were perceived as "friendly", "cheerful" and "welcoming". However, this was counter-balanced by smaller, though significant proportions of mothers who described the environment as "strict", "frightening", "depressing" and "impersonal". The busy atmosphere also concerned some, as did the rules and regulations they felt imposed on them.

Table 9.7 · The most frequent positive and negative adjectives chosen by mothers to describe the atmosphere in the neonatal unit. (n=418 mothers)

		Adjectives used			
		Positive	**%**	**Negative**	**%**
Rank	1	Friendly	81.7	Hectic	28.6
	2	Cheerful	71.4	Strict	18.3
	3	Welcoming	68.8	Frightening	11.4
	4	Efficient	67.1	Impersonal	10.0
	5	Organised	66.7	Depressing	8.8

Involvement in Care

For parents separation is the worst and most painful aspect of having a baby admitted to a neonatal unit:

> 'I was separated from my baby. Not able to hold her she did not feel like my baby.'

> 'When I had to leave my baby at night and when I was discharged it was terrible. I didn't want to leave him behind. I cried every night.'

> 'The worst thing was being worried if she was alright, and not being able to be with her all the time.'

Linked with the experience of separation is the loss of role and identity as a parent. Protecting and caring for your baby is an essential element in parenting and yet, at least early on, many parents were unable or felt unable to take on this very basic aspect of the role:

> 'I had to ask advice all the time. I felt like she wasn't my baby and someone else had taken over her care and I was just a bystander.'

> 'I was unable to stay with him so I didn't see anything they did to him in my absence. I was frightened that something might happen to him when I wasn't there.'

> 'The worst thing was not caring for her the way I wanted to and knowing she was solely dependant on the nurses and not me as her mother.'

Facilitating contact and involving parents' in their baby's care is thought to be an important method of overcoming the emotional problems that can arise in the short-term and of avoiding some of the longer term consequences of separation (Klaus and Kennell,1982). The stage at which mothers and their partners first saw, touched and held their babies is shown in Figure 9.4. Many parents touched and held their babies early on, but a small proportion did not have this kind of contact until somewhat later. Even those who did have this contact were keenly aware of what having your baby cared for in this type of environment meant:

> 'I felt like she wasn't really mine, I always had to ask if I could do this or that for her.'

> 'I could not touch my baby unless they said I could'

> 'Not being able to hold our baby, I felt as though I was being watched all the time.'

> 'I did not feel he was my baby and felt I had to ask before I could do anything. This was my feeling and not the hospital.'

The "milestones" of participating and taking over the care of your baby are very important ones to both parents. This is especially true when progress is slow

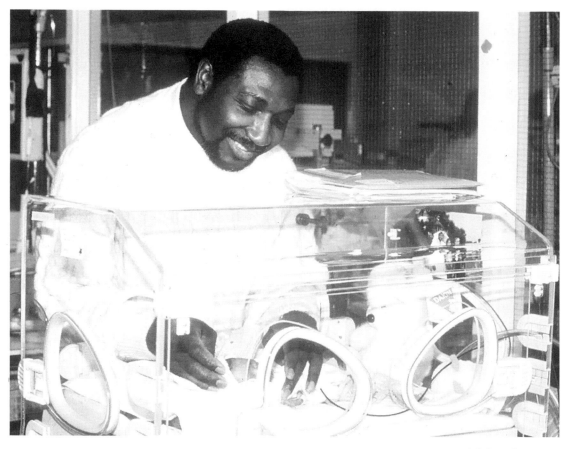

A father enjoys getting involved in the care of his small baby

and babies are in hospital for some time. The time point at which mothers became involved in active care for their baby is show in Figure 9.5. A shift can be seen over the items, with some mothers increasingly taking over more of the caretaking tasks from the nurses. Units and individual members of staff differed in the extent to which they were willing to encourage parents, though official policy in general was aimed at helping the development of parenting skills. Parents also differed and some had ambivalent feelings about their baby's care and their own competence. Fear and anxiety may make it difficult to respond in the way staff expected them to and to follow their advice.

TIMING OF FIRST CONTACT

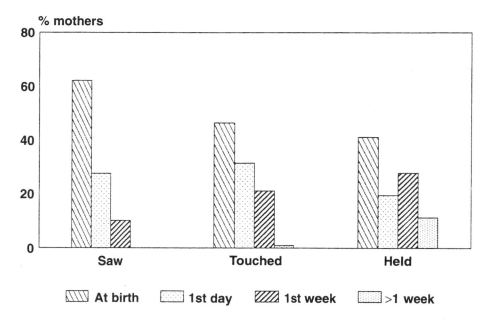

Figure 9.4a · Stage at which mothers first saw, touched and held their babies (n=420 mothers)

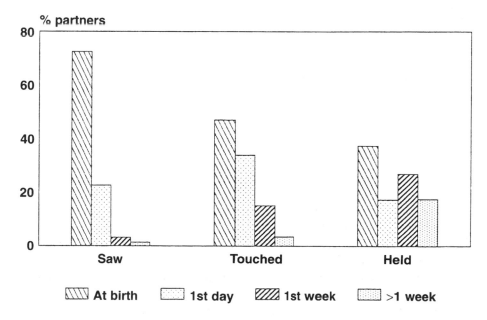

Figure 9.4b · Stage at which partners first saw, touched and held their babies (n=390 partners)

MOTHERS' INVOLVEMENT IN CARE

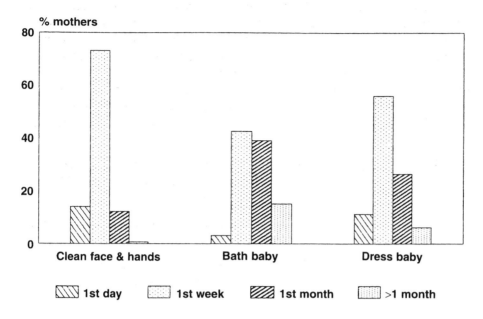

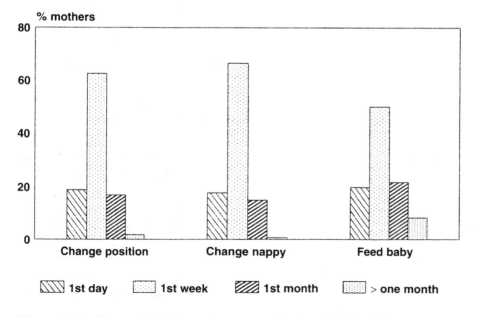

Figure 9.5 · Stage at which mothers were first involved in different aspects of infant care (n=420 mothers)

Feeding is one of the most important aspects of care in which parents, particularly mothers can be directly involved (Ingram et al, 1994). Of the study babies admitted to neonatal care 37% were fed intravenously at some time, usually early on in their stay. More than half the mothers (55%) expressed their own breast milk and looked forward to this being given to their baby in the form of a tube feed. Actually carrying out the tube feeding, whether using expressed breast milk or formula, was a task that many mothers were keen to carry out and 52% did so at some time, though in some units this was not allowed at all. The problem of timing also arose in relation to important events like feeds, that are seen as "firsts" by parents:

'I was upset about not having control over decisions about her care. Her first oral feed was given without consultation whereas I would have liked to have been the first to feed her this way.'

Also, not fitting in with parents' visiting can reduce their sense of control and involvement:

'We liked to visit the hospital at least twice a day after I was discharged to feed Harry. We found it most annoying and hurtful when we arrived and the nurses had already done it early or altered the times without phoning us.'

A number of mothers were also concerned that their babies were being tube fed to save the nurses' time and that this was not for the baby's benefit:

'When feeding a prem baby they drink slowly, but if the baby hasn't drunk it in 10 minutes, the nurses put it down the tube. Jenny takes 40 minutes to drink six oz of milk. Prem babies need a lot of time for their food.'

'Simon took the bottle happily from me, but the nurses insisted on tube-feeding. Presumably its quicker, but no satisfactory explanation was given.'

Moving on to breast or bottle feeding was also seen as an important step. A total of 49% of mothers breastfed or tried to breastfeed while their baby was in the neonatal unit; at discharge the proportion breastfeeding was 31% and at the time of the questionnaire, sent out at two months post-discharge, 14% were still feeding this way. All the study mothers were asked about advice, help and assistance with feeding. Their views are summarised in Table 9.8. (Some mothers both breast and bottle fed their babies while in the neonatal units and so have given their views about both forms of feeding). The impression given by mothers and directly from visiting the units is that though efforts are being made in this area, more could be done:

'I was not given the choice at the time to express milk or not. Formula milk was already being given.'

'They were very busy and this meant mothers were not given as much help and advice as we needed.'

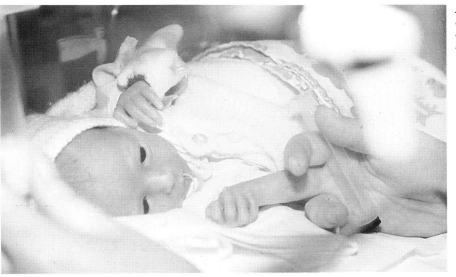

A small baby who is alert and responsive after being tube-fed by her mother

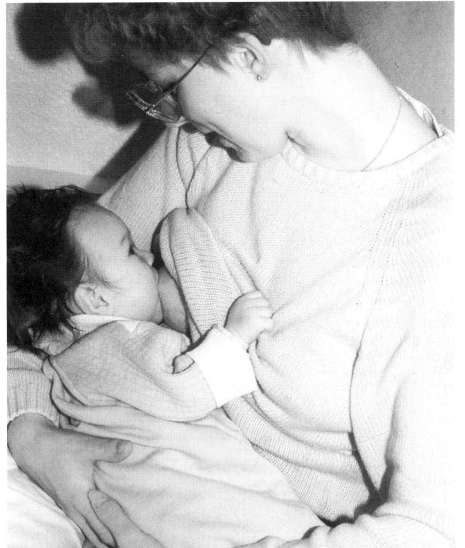

A mother breast feeding in neonatal care

Table 9.8 · The availability of assistance in neonatal units with different aspects of breastfeeding and bottle feeding

	% Mothers	
	Breastfeeding n=214	**Bottle feeding** n=318
Insufficient		
Advice	32.7	39.0
Practical help	31.8	33.3
Active support and encouragement	29.9	42.4
Explanation of how feeding works	43.0	48.7
Privacy to feed	34.6	34.3

'Over the first few days I had to ask if I could put him to the breast. I think they assumed that I would just express and sort out breast feeding later. If I was a first time mum, or younger, I wouldn't have had the confidence to put baby to the breast when I did. As it was, he took to it very well.'

The need for privacy while expressing and feeding was an issue commented on by many mothers.

'It is not easy expressing, especially at first. There was nowhere to express that was private.'

'Whilst trying to breast feed there was no privacy and a very limited amount of room to put screens around.'

'I felt there wasn't enough privacy while trying to breast feed. Men mending equipment were in and out, also porters, nurses, doctors and other families with babies in SCBU.'

'I did not mind feeding her with doctors and nurses present, but felt rather uncomfortable in front of other parents.'

Of the twenty-four units visited, only two had a comfortable breast feeding room specifically for that purpose, that was not a cupboard, kitchen, shared part of a sitting room or corner of a laboratory. Expressing took place in a variety of similar locations, though slightly more privacy was provided for this activity. The use of small or inadequate screens was noted at a number of sites.

Involvement of other family members, especially siblings and grandparents is thought to be important (McHaffie, 1992) when babies are admitted to intensive care. Single parents with a baby in a neonatal unit feel particularly vulnerable and the support that can come from close family members or friends is much needed. Visiting policies varied between units; all the twenty-four studied allowed open visiting for parents, but there were often restrictions of some sort for other children, friends and relatives. Of those families with other children, most siblings were allowed to visit, but for 19 families (4%) this was not allowed. The majority (86%) of babies were visited by at least one grandparent, though for 33% of families other relatives were not allowed in the neonatal unit. Friends were less likely to be allowed to visit, even accompanying parents. Relatively few units had a policy which referred to parents' choice of "significant others" rather than family members.

The degree to which parents felt involved in the care of their baby and the degree to which they could be involved, obviously depended upon many factors including the condition of the baby and their own attitudes. However, the differences in policy between units and the different rules in operation can only have complicated and exacerbated the problems that can arise in adjusting to being the parent of "a special care baby".

The Need For Information

The need for information is a paramount one in the medical and technological context of care today (Audit Commission, 1993a). Many parents with a baby in neonatal care were aware of their own information needs:

> 'The worst thing was not being told why she was in, what their diagnosis was, what happened in labour, and whether she would be OK or not.'

> 'I was not in any way prepared for giving birth to a "poorly" baby. Ante-natal classes did not cover this at all. The birth itself was not how I had envisaged it and I would have welcomed more support and explanation as to Sam's condition.'

On being asked to comment on their personal experience and what they could draw from it that could be of help to other parents, the need to seek information was emphasised:

> 'Don't hesitate to ask the staff if there is anything you don't understand – even if they are very busy, wait for an explanation, rather than leaving the unit worrying.'

> 'Ask as many questions as possible and nag at the doctors and nurses, because if you don't, they will not tell you anything.'

> 'Never be afraid to ask about your babies problems and treatment.'

The neonatal unit staff are a key resource for parents needing information and support. How they were used by parents while their baby was in the neonatal unit is shown in Table 9.9. From this it is evident the nursing and medical staff in many instances provided a great deal of help: doctors, both junior and senior, predominantly gave information; nurses also gave explanations and advice but

Table 9.9 · The proportions of parents receiving different kinds of help from different sources within the neonatal unit (n=420)

Sources of Help	Type of Help			
	Explanations	Advice	Support	Sympathy
Senior doctors	61.5	22.5	18.7	10.8
Junior doctors	42.2	23.9	16.7	11.0
Senior nurses	69.8	65.1	57.7	35.1
Junior nurses	52.0	55.4	59.9	38.7
Other parents	5.6	11.0	33.8	23.6
Social worker	3.6	4.7	5.9	3.6
Support group	0.9	2.3	2.7	1.6
Religious advisor	0.2	0.5	4.3	3.8

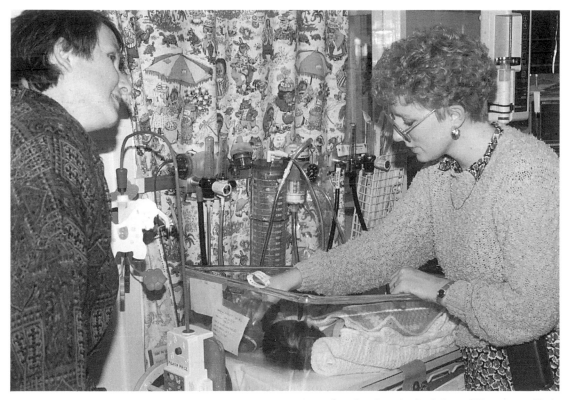

A mother discussing her baby and his progress with the unit social worker

additionally functioned as sources of support and sympathy. A third of parents also used other parents as a source of support. Social workers, support groups and religious advisors were relatively little used at this stage.

Neonatal unit staff, though they are the main channel for information, are often busy. Parents do not always feel able to ask questions and information is sometimes better understood when presented in more than one form. A checklist was made at each unit visit of what information actually was available for parents and a summary shown in Table 9.10.

Overall, there seems to have been a slowness to take on board and acknowledge parents' need for information. That less than half the units had their own information booklet and that the same proportion had no booklet at all, would suggest this aspect of care is not taken as seriously as it might be. Being able to identify staff by name and role within the unit is another aspect of providing information, but without photo-boards this is difficult. The variable use of badges, some of which say only "Auntie Pat" or "Sister" did nothing to make the identification easier for parents. The advent of "the named nurse" may have facilitated an improvement in this area (Hancock, 1992; DOH, 1993).

Gaining access to medical information concerning their baby can also be difficult on some units. In 75% (18), parents were allowed to stay for ward rounds but in the remainder they were asked to leave the room. For a variety of reasons many parents feel inhibited from asking questions and excluding some in this way may constrain them further. A more flexible arrangement that could satisfy parents' needs and ethical problems for staff may be for parents to be

Table 9.10 · Sources of written or visual information for parents in the neonatal units studied

| | Unit Type | | | |
	Regional (n=6)	Subregional (n=6)	District (n=12)	Total (n=24)
Notice About Visiting	3	4	9	16
No Booklet	1	5	4	10
Own Booklet	5	1	4	10
Booklet produced by Baby Food Manufacturer	–	–	4	4
Information Board used, with:	5	6	8	19
Staff Names	3	4	5	12
Staff Photos	3	4	6	13
Previous Babies' Photos	5	6	9	20
Parent Group Contact	4	4	6	14
Statutory Services Leaflets	4	5	6	15

included and hear what is said about their own baby but not to be present during discussions about other babies.

Parents in general can find it hard to understand the exact nature of their baby's problems and the medical equipment and procedures used:

> 'I was upset and said I couldn't really understand why he had to be there. But we were made to feel welcome and then each monitor and drug used was explained that day and again another time.'

> 'I was overwhelmed with everything going on, and found it hard to understand what all the tubes and monitors were used for.'

It seems that consistent advice and more information is needed in different formats to suit the wide range of parents whose babies are admitted to neonatal units. However, despite the gaps, at least in retrospect, most of the study parents had a positive view of the extent to which their baby's problems and the associated medical equipment had been explained (Figure 9.6). Parents' perceptions of the wide range of procedures carried out on their baby in neonatal care varied. Of the babies having specific procedures of which the parents were aware, the proportions that were worried by these are shown in Table 9.11.

Parents of sick babies receiving complex treatment are likely to be anxious and worried about what is happening to their baby. However, both they, and

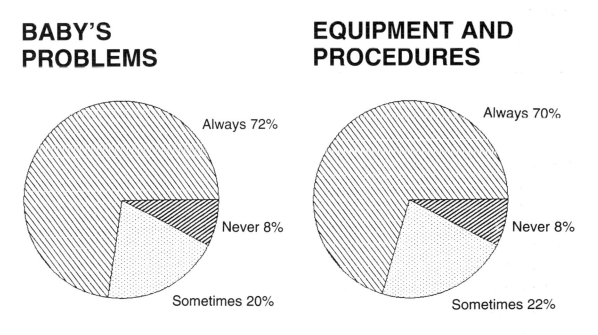

BABY'S PROBLEMS

Always 72%

Never 8%

Sometimes 20%

EQUIPMENT AND PROCEDURES

Always 70%

Never 8%

Sometimes 22%

Figure 9.6 · Frequency of explanations given to parents about different aspects of their baby's care (n=420)

Table 9.11 · The proportions of babies having specific medical procedures in neonatal care and the proportions of parents that were worried by these procedures

Medical Procedure	% Babies Having Procedure	% Parents Worried
A heel-prick blood sample	94.4	56.5
Feeding tube in the nose or mouth	90.3	68.1
Blood sample taken from arm or leg	62.4	64.6
IV drip in arm of leg	57.8	81.4
Injection	51.4	50.9
An X-ray	52.9	43.4
Wires on chest for monitoring	47.8	50.5
Eye shields and phototherapy	45.5	32.7
Breathing tube in the nose or mouth	30.2	82.1
Suction tube used to clear secretions	30.2	64.7
Splints to restrain arms or legs	28.4	63.5
Ultra-sound scan of baby's head	27.5	69.7
Blood transfusion	23.0	82.4
IV drip attached to baby's head	14.6	95.4
Blood sample taken through a catheter	14.4	57.8
Chest drain	6.8	90.0

parents with babies having less serious problems, may feel different when they understand more about the procedures and the reasons for carrying them out. Just because in medical or nursing terms a procedure is trivial or routine it cannot be assumed that it is not perceived as important by the parents:

> 'The worst thing was all the equipment around and the incubator flashing and beeping away.'

> 'I hated her being under the phototherapy light – she looked so wretched.'

> 'Her poor heels were red raw from heel pricks.'

A great deal of unnecessary anxiety could be saved by staff being more aware and acknowledging the concerns of parents in this area. That so many parents were worried about nasogastric tubes, heel-pricks and blood samples illustrates this point. With the more serious invasive procedures perhaps time needs to be taken on more than one occasion to talk to parents about these. Where staff perceived and responded to the need in this area, parents recognised the value of this kind of input and were very appreciative:

> 'The staff were so kind and good in explaining the procedures to my partner and myself and answering all our questions.'

> 'The best thing was a caring and optimistic midwife who had the time to talk and discuss my baby's problems'

Examination of parents' responses as a whole shows that the three areas where information is most needed are: on the medical procedures and equipment, on feeding, and on their own feelings at this time. In addition to the verbal explanations from the neonatal staff a unit booklet, posters, a small library, parent contacts and an experienced health care worker (health visitor, social worker or psychologist) available on a regular sessional basis, could do much to answer these needs.

The Environment and Facilities

The physical surroundings of the neonatal unit environment can affect both staff and parents. A checklist was used during the unit visits and a summary of items recorded is shown in Table 9.12.

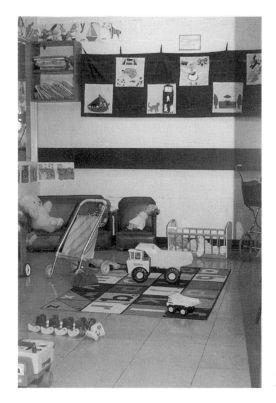

A specifically designed play area for visiting children

Table 9.12 · Features of neonatal units visited (n=24 units)

		Type of Unit			
		Regional (n=6)	Subregional (n=6)	District (n=12)	Total (n=24)
Entrance area	Gloomy	3	4	3	10
	Bright	2	2	2	6
	Neutral	1	1	6	8
Access	Ring Bell/Wait	4	5	8	17
	Walk in	2	1	4	7
Unit	Gloomy	1	3	3	7
	Bright	3	3	9	15
	Neutral	2	–	–	2
Decoration/ furnishings	Curtains/Blinds	6	6	11	23
	Wallpaper	1	4	6	11
	Easy Chairs	6	5	9	20
	Pictures	5	4	9	18
	Mobiles	4	3	10	17
	Stickers	5	6	8	19
	Cards	3	4	4	11
Accommodation For families	Sitting Room	5	6	11	22
	Overnight for Mother	6	6	9	21
	Overnight for Both Parents	6	6	9	21

With the advent of "family centred care" most units are making efforts to make the whole environment more parent-friendly and welcoming, but a smaller number were making only limited efforts in this direction. In these there was clearly room for improvement. Motivation seemed to be a factor here as the kind of features listed are possible at relatively low cost, in comparison with the expense involved, for example, in buying technical equipment.

Parents and staff working in the same units were asked about aspects of the physical environment and where improvements were required (Table 9.13). Nursing staff working in neonatal care were apparently more critical or more aware of the deficits than the parents. While parents may be overwhelmed or preoccupied with their baby, nurses who work in these units over a long period of time have greater exposure to the environmental problems. Nevertheless, parents did mention cramped conditions, heating and air conditioning problems and inadequate furnishings.

'The rooms were so cramped there was hardly any space to put the screen for feeding, and no room for visitors.'

Table 9.13 · A comparison of parents and nursing staff views on the physical environment of the neonatal unit (n=420 parents, 718 nurses)

Improvements Needed	% Parents	% Nursing staff
Space	53.8	68.7
Noise	13.1	49.4
Temperature	19.9	61.1
Air-conditioning	35.8	73.7
Humidity	30.2	58.8
Decoration	14.9	42.3
Furnishings	25.2	59.4
Lighting	8.6	51.5

'In the other hospital there was no cooled water supply and in that heat you really needed it.'

'There were very few comfortable chairs you could sit in and cuddle your baby.'

In summary it seems that a pleasant environment, in which staff and parents feel comfortable working and caring for babies is likely to encourage a positive attitude on the part of both. The chronic lack of space in many units, the use of corridors as storerooms and shared accommodation for parents and staff makes them both feel less valued and cared for. Only seven of the twenty-four study units were modern and purpose-built for neonatal care and even these were not free of the kind of problems mentioned.

Transfer and its Consequences for Parents and Families

Access to and availability of specialist services in a number of areas, including neonatal intensive care, has been the focus of a report by the Clinical Standards Advisory Group (CSAG, 1993). One in five of the babies in the study (88 of 444) were transferred to at least one other unit able to provide more long term intensive care or with a facility for neonatal surgery. Some (14%) were cared for in just one other unit, though 6% of babies experienced care in three or more different hospitals before being discharged home.

For parents the key issues arising from transfers of their "sick" infant are those associated with reduced proximity and separation, confidence in care and communication. Problems associated with these issues can arise at each stage in the transfer process: during the initial decision-making; concerning the nature of the transfer itself; in the course of staying in and visiting the hospital to which their baby has been moved and then in transferring back to the home unit. The fears and anxieties can be exacerbated by the need for transfer and parents, though to some extent reassured, may feel ambivalent about their baby's move to a specialist centre:

'I was just so shocked at him being taken away from us'

'The hospital she was transferred to was good, but so far away'

Delays in decision-making, problems in finding a cot in a referral unit and arranging transport all affect parents:

'It was terrible knowing he needed the care and waiting for a cot to be found'

'We were upset at being left behind while he was rushed without us to the big baby unit'

The idea of their baby being sent off into the unknown is distressing for most parents in this situation and being informed about the need for transfer, the personnel involved and the arrangements are important at this critical time. The development of a more coordinated approach and of transport teams specifically for neonatal care (Leslie and Stephenson, 1994; Macrae, 1994) will undoubtedly contribute positively in this respect.

Information about the referral centre itself is also valued by parents:

'It helped to be told about the hospital my baby was going to for her operation'

'The nurses showed us some pictures of where he was going and gave us a leaflet about the special care baby unit there'

Once their baby has been transferred to another unit other problems can arise. Twins and babies from multiple births may be split up and parents can feel really torn with their babies being cared for in different hospitals. Visiting and staying in the transfer hospital can also be problematic: parents are often isolated from their partner, from other children and their wider family, as well as separated from the baby. In the larger units the environment may be more technological; there are also different staff; there may be different rules and expectations of parents and the travel requirements can disrupt family life considerably:

'I felt lost, it was so high-tech and so much equipment'

'Being in a big city, miles from home, the hospital became our base, but we still felt lonely'

'Our family and friends couldn't visit because of the distance'

'We were both worn out with the worry and the travelling'

Transferring back to the local unit, though nearer to home, was not always straightforward. Limited contact and liaison between units, variations in practice and concern about local unit staff skills and the equipment available were evident:

> 'The rules were different in our local baby unit, and I got told off for not doing things right.'

> 'I felt worried about leaving my baby after he was transferred back from the big SCBU.'

> 'We didn't feel so confident about the way they cared for her when she came back'

However, there were clear benefits to being transferred back to a unit near home:

> 'It was nice to have our baby back in the local hospital where the staff seemed to have more time for us.'

> 'I needed my Mum and after the baby came back to our local hospital she could visit and help with his care'

Moving babies from one unit to another affects parents directly and their relationships with the local hospital health care professionals on whom their baby's care will depend in the future. Agreed policies and standards, close and regular contact between units where transfers are common and regular communication concerning individual babies and their families may ameliorate many of the difficulties experienced by parents in this area. Other positive measures such as staff exchanges, outreach schemes, booklets about the different units and photograph albums also contribute. On the practical side, the provision of adequate overnight accommodation for both parents and play facilities for siblings, can make a considerable difference to families travelling some distance. While some "model" units might have some or all of what is suggested and provide examples of "good practice", there are still large inter-unit differences which imply that there is considerable room for change in addressing the needs of families in this situation.

Bereaved Parents

Bereaved parents are a special group that it was felt important to include within the study. They represent a minority of the parents of babies cared for in neonatal units, and yet in improving the way that they are cared for, much has also been done to enhance the awareness of parents' experiences in general.

A total of 19 families whose babies had died were recruited to the study. Their babies had been cared for in one or more of the study units for at least two days. Of these families 14 agreed to participate and 12 (63%) returned completed questionnaires. The details of the babies are as follows: five of the twelve babies were boys and seven were girls; seven were preterm and five were born at term and they had been cared for in seven different neonatal units (five regional and two subregional centres).

For the purposes of comparing the way that parents whose baby died may have experienced neonatal care with that of families with surviving infants, matched controls were obtained from the main study. These were matched as closely as possible on gestational age, birthweight, sex, mother's age, type of unit and the presence of an abnormality. Details of means and ranges on birthweight and gestational age for the two groups are shown in Table 9.14. Other details of the two groups are shown in Table 9.15. No significant differences were found between the groups on the aspects listed.

Table 9.14 · A comparison of the birthweights and gestational ages of the matched groups of babies

		Babies who died	Control Babies
Gestational Age at Birth (weeks)	Mean	32.2	32.4
	Range	24–40	26–42
Birthweight (kg)	Mean	1.90	1.94
	Range	690g-3.57	640g-3.54

Table 9.15 · A comparison of the experiences and background of the bereaved and control group mothers

	Mothers of Babies who died (n=12)	Control Mothers (n=12)
Partner	12	11
Other Children	7	5
Under School Age Children	8	3
Antenatal Stay	7	5
In Utero Transfer	4	3
Caesarean Section Delivery	4	1
Baby Transferred	4	2
Previous Baby in SCBU	3	2
Seen the Unit Antenally	1	2

A summary of the facilities available for parents whose baby has died in the 24 hospitals visited is shown in Table 9.16.

Table 9.16 · The facilities available for bereaved parents in different types of neonatal unit

	Unit Type			
	Regional (n=6)	Subregional (n=6)	District (n=12)	Total (n=24)
Quiet Room	5	6	2	13
Small Crib or Cot	6	6	12	24
A Bereavement Booklet (SANDS)	4	5	11	20
Other Information	3	4	4	11
Consultant Follow-up	6	6	11	23

A comparison of parental concerns on first seeing their infant in neonatal care is shown in Table 9.17. Both groups were equally concerned about how their baby looked and the monitor noise, though more bereaved parents subsequently referred more to the equipment and what a nurse had said at this stage.

Table 9.17 · Aspects of the neonatal care situation that concerned bereaved and control parents when they first saw their baby

Aspects of Neonatal Care	Bereaved Parents (n=12)	Control Parents (n=12)
Equipment	10	5
Baby's appearance	7	7
Noise	6	6
Temperature	2	3
Busy atmosphere	2	2
What doctor said	6	4
What nurse said	5	0

Involvement in their baby's care was less frequent for the bereaved parents, probably as a result of the baby's condition. All the bereaved mothers and partners had seen and touched their baby while he or she was alive, though in only 7 of the 12 cases did they hold and cuddle their baby at this stage. More than half had undertaken their baby's "cares" and changed a nappy, but fewer had fed their baby.

No significant difference was found between the groups concerning the adequacy of the explanations given and discussion of their baby's problems and the technical equipment in use. Almost all of the bereaved parents (11 out of

12) felt that the equipment and procedures were always explained to them and that their baby's problems were discussed fully with them (10 out of 12). Both groups of parents had similar concerns about the physical environment of neonatal care and indicated from their perspective that the lack of space and cramped conditions required improvement. The need for privacy was also an issue for both groups. At this point more of the bereaved parents (5 out of 12 compared with 1 out of 12) again referred to the noise of alarms and monitors.

In terms of the atmosphere in the unit the bereaved parents were as positive as the controls. None of them perceived it as impersonal, strict or disorganised and more than three-quarters described the atmosphere as "friendly", "welcoming", "efficient" and "reassuring". However, one family experienced the unit as "hostile" at times, another as "depressing" and two as "frightening". That bereaved parents sometimes focused on the more mechanistic and intrusive aspects of neonatal care is not surprising in the context of this highly technical environment and with their personal experience of having had only limited time and contact with their baby.

All but one of the families were with their baby when he or she died. Afterwards all the parents held their baby and half of them took part in bathing and dressing the baby. A third took their other children or close relatives to see the baby at this time.

Of 56 units in the first stage of the study, 23 (41%) reported that a bereavement counsellor was available and in 21 (38%) the Registrar of births and deaths visited the hospital. Summaries of the facilities used by the study parents after their baby died and the staff they saw is contained in Tables 9.18. and 9.19. The bereaved parents felt they were treated well and sympathetically but they also had comments to make. The emphasis in these was on the need for better communication and honesty, the need to be listened to and not hurried:

Table 9.18 · Facilities and services used by bereaved parents (n=12)

Facilities and services used			
Quiet room to be with baby	11	Help with funeral arrangements	6
Baptism, blessing or ceremony	3	Leaflets written for bereaved parents	10
Crib or moses basket	9	Parent support group information (SANDS)	8
Photographs	10	Babies' book of remembrance	3
Keepsakes (name band)	11	Service of remembrance	2

Table 9.19 · People that bereaved parents talked to in the month after the baby died (n=12)

People talked to			
Consultant paediatrician	6	Registrar of deaths	11
Pathologist	0	Midwife/Health visitor	9
Nursing staff	6	GP	10
Clergy	7	Bereavement counsellor	2
Social worker	3	Psychologist	1

'At the end of Joanna's life we felt pressurised and rushed to make the decision to turn off the machines. I felt terrible. Parents need to take time to make decisions and should not be put on the spot to decide there and then.'

'When we were told he would die, they told us very quickly and then the consultant jumped quickly to saying that I had another baby (his twin.)'

'Because they switched the machines off, the staff were all aware of the situation. Some avoided us and others didn't know what to say. It was uncomfortable for us, as well as upsetting.'

'I felt that the doctors could have been more honest. They would not commit themselves to tell me when things were definitely not looking very good, and my son was actually dying.'

'Doctors need to explain things more clearly to parents rather than them having to ask.'

The enforcement of visiting rules upset one family:

'I would have liked my sister to see my daughter. She was not allowed in the room, but saw her through glass. I think this should be changed. My family are a close-knit unit and are very loving and I was disappointed.'

An important point which applies in neonatal care as a whole was made by a mother:

'Doctors, nurses, the health visitor, friends, all asked me how I felt, but not so much her father. I got nearly all the sympathy, advice and explanations, even though her Dad was suffering her loss as much as me.'

Supporting parents whose baby is dying or has died requires expertise, sensitivity and awareness of the needs of parents (Gustaitis and Young, 1986).

Neonatal nurses, even under pressure, provide much of this, but support and training at all levels is needed, both for them to care for parents and to be able to work through their own feelings as carers.

> 'I had to inform parents that their 12 hour old son's condition had deteriorated and when they came, support them as the doctors told them that the baby was not going to survive and that ventilation should be withdrawn. I was with them when their baby died.'

> 'A 'chronic' baby died who'd been on the unit for over five months. No one talked about it and I was close to his parents. I went to the funeral and after the service other colleagues also there disappeared quickly, leaving me to go back with the family. Since then no one has asked how I feel and nobody has offered any support whatsoever. It has been left to non-nursing friends to pick me up and encourage me to stick at neonatal nursing.'

It seems that a more perceptive and in many instances a more structured approach to the immediate and longer term needs of both parents and staff is required in this area.

Parent Care: Holistic or Realistic?

On the whole it seems that parents make the best of what is for them a difficult time. In retrospect, most were grateful to the nursing and medical staff for the care that their baby had received. They may not have been aware of staffing or equipment shortages or skill mix problems, but this does not mean they were uncritical of certain aspects of neonatal care.

Neonatal nursing as a profession is moving in the direction of a philosophy of care in which the whole family is considered. The responses of parents indicate that a more parent and family-oriented approach is in the process of slowly being adopted. Treating parents as individuals and responding to their needs in an individual way, is agreed to be important, but in practice inflexible rules and policies and different interpretations of these, often prevent this. For many of the families with a baby admitted to neonatal care, there has already been disruption to family life before the birth and this, in conjunction with relatively high levels of obstetric intervention, puts them at a further disadvantage when compared with mothers delivering normally and caring for their baby during a short stay on a postnatal ward (Keirse, 1989).

As in other areas of paediatrics, there can be conflict between the need to address parents' needs individually and as a group, and nursing or medical priorities (Audit Commission, 1993b). Though the baby is officially "the patient" in the context of neonatal care, the neonatal unit is only a temporary home and the needs of the whole family require consideration and planning from the time of admission and in some cases before delivery. The importance of keeping in touch with parents' perceptions of their baby's condition and care is difficult to over-emphasise. With bereaved parents for whom the neonatal unit is commonly their baby's only home, many nursing staff feel the weight of the responsibility in trying to care for these families:

> 'I was caring for a dying baby and performing last offices. Despite feeling quite confident about the procedures, I felt inadequate in dealing with the baby's parents and relatives. I performed my duties adequately yet still felt unable to do anything constructive. I was trying to be supportive to the baby's family, yet experiencing grief myself and feeling so helpless – knowing there was nothing I could do except be a comforting presence.'

In any unit it is necessary to create and maintain a climate in which parental access is encouraged and facilitated (Thornes, 1984). As parents of a sick or small baby they need a safe and comfortable place in which their own and their baby's needs are recognised and in which they are able to make a relationship with their baby (Redshaw et al, 1994). This is despite the unusual environment, their baby's medical problems, limited access and control and their own intense anxiety and uncertainty. This means having staff sensitive to the needs of individuals under stress in an unexpectedly dependent relationship, with sufficient time to talk, explain and listen. Many parents are involved in the care of their baby and the extent to which this occurs varies, sometimes as a function of the baby's condition, but also due to other factors. A need for written policies that are clear and accessible to all members of staff and parents is evident in most units. The broader need for parents to have information is poorly addressed for the most part: information should be presented in a variety of formats, and not simply as one small booklet or display on a notice board (Alderson, 1983).

In caring for parents, as in other aspects of neonatal care, there are differences in policy, attitudes, organisation and practice that give rise to examples of good practice and less good practice. Even in units with well-thought out and clearly stated philosophies of care, there were gaps between these and their implementation in care and organisation. The findings from the present study of parents and units in many parts of England indicate areas in which progress has been made (Brimblecombe et al, 1978; Davis et al, 1983) and where more effort is required. Addressing the medical, practical and psychosocial needs of the whole family and translating "holistic family care" into a reality is a difficult task and a challenge for the future on which most units are just beginning to focus.

References

Alderson, P. (1983) Special Care for Babies in Hospital. National Association for the Welfare of Children in Hospital, London.

Audit Commission, (1993a) What Seems to be the Matter: Communication between Hospitals and Patients. HMSO, London.

Audit Commission, (1993b) Children First: Improving the Health Care of Sick Children, HMSO, London.

Brimblecombe, F., Richards, M. and Roberton, N. (1978) Separation and special care baby units, Clinics in Developmental Medicine, 68. Heineman, London.

de Chateau, P. and Wiberg, B. (1984) Long-term effect on mother–infant behaviour of extra contact during the first hour post-partum. *Scandinavian Journal of Social Medicine*, **12**, 91–103.

Clinical Standards Advisory Group (1993) Access and Availability of Specialist Services. DOH, HMSO London.

Davis, J. A., Richards, M. P. M. and Roberton, N. R. C.(1983) Parent-baby Attachment in Premature Infants. London, Croom Helm.

Department of Health (1993) A Vision for the Future. DOH/NHSME, London.

Greene J. G., Fox N. A. and Lewis, M. (1983). The relationship between neonatal characteristics and three-month mother-infant interaction in high-risk infants. *Child Development*, **54**, 1286–1296.

Gustaitis, R. and Young, E. W. D. (1986). A Time to be Born and a Time to Die: Conflicts and Ethics in an Intensive Care Unit. Addison Wesley, Reading, Massachusetts.

Hancock, C. (1992) The named nurse concept. *Nursing Standard*, **6**, 17.

Ingram, J., Redshaw, M. and Harris, A. (1994) Breastfeeding in neonatal care. *British Journal of Midwifery*, **2**, 412–418.

Jeffcoate, J. A., Humphrey, M. E. and Lloyd, J. K. (1979) Disturbances in parent-child relationship following preterm delivery. *Developmental Medicine and Child Neurology*, **21**, 344–352.

Keirse, M. (1989) Preterm delivery. Chapter in Effective Care in Pregnancy and Childbirth, 2, Eds. Chalmers, Enkin and Keirse, Oxford University Press, Oxford. 1270–1292.

Klaus, M. H. and Kennell, J. H. (1982) Parent-Infant Bonding. St Louis, C.V. Mosby.

Leslie, A. and Stephenson, T. (1994) Audit of neonatal intensive care transport. *Archives of Disease in Childhood*. **71**, F61-F66.

Macrae, D. J. (1994) Paediatric intensive care transport. *Archives of Disease in Childhood*. **71**, 175–178.

McHaffie, Hazel E. (1989) Mothers of very low birthweight babies: who supports them? *Midwifery* **5**, 113–121.

McHaffie, Hazel E. (1990) Mothers of very low birthweight babies: How do they adjust? *Journal of Advanced Nursing*. **15**, 6–11.

McHaffie, Hazel E. (1992), Social support in the neonatal intensive care unit. *Journal of Advanced Nursing*, **17**, 279–287.

Redshaw, M. E., Rivers, R. P. A. and Rosenblatt, D. B. (1985). Born Too Early. Special care for your preterm baby. Oxford University Press, Oxford.

Redshaw, M. E., Harris, A. and Ingram, J. C. (1994) A Home from Home ? Policy and practice as it affects parents with a baby in neonatal care. *Child Health*, **2**, 79–84.

The Royal College of Physicians, (1988). Medical Care of The Newborn in England and Wales. RCP, London.

Thornes, R. (1984) Parental Access and Family Facilities in Special and Intensive Care Neonatal Units in England. Unpublished Report, National Association for the Welfare of Children in Hospital, London.

Chapter 10 · Directions for the Future

Issues and Implications

The picture gained in the course of the present study is of neonatal nurses under pressure, which at times is extreme. Many nurses working in neonatal units feel they are just getting by on a day-to-day basis: patient care may be the last thing to suffer, but in the meantime, the individuals and the service count the cost. The stresses and psychological wear and tear that come from the nature of the job itself are exacerbated by organisational problems and staffing difficulties as well as personal factors. Effective team-work and mutual support are difficult to maintain in these circumstances, but are essential if nurses are to want to stay in the specialty.

While the last two decades have seen the situation improve for sick babies and their families, less attention has been focused on the staff who care for them. Much change and innovation in this area is envisaged if the issues raised directly and indirectly in the course of this study are to be addressed. In neonatal nursing, as in nursing generally, a change is needed in the attitude to nurses as working women, many of whom have the responsibilities of families and dependents. The evidence is that they are an integral part of the workforce and should be seen as a valuable resource to be utilised, rather than as a hindrance to better organisation. Older, experienced nurses too are a resource to be valued, but in this fast-changing technically-oriented specialty, their situation requires discussion and planning; simply promoting or down-grading them is not sufficient. The question of professional development is also one to be faced, with professional bodies, managers at different levels and motivated nurses needing to work together. Better and more appropriate management training for senior nurses could be used as a means of facilitating further change: with promotion comes the title, but not the skills that go with the position. The development of the role of nurse managers as leaders for change in the neonatal unit is an important one, but only as a part of a team where nurses, support workers and medical staff are considered to be active elements and contributors as well.

The commonly felt demoralisation that goes with not being able to meet both the demands and professional standards, indicates that the problems of the neonatal unit as a working environment are widespread. Neonatal units are not constructed with "elastic walls", budgets are limited and hospitals are competing with one another. As the personnel most continually in the neonatal unit and with the greatest contact with the client group, nursing staff have been the

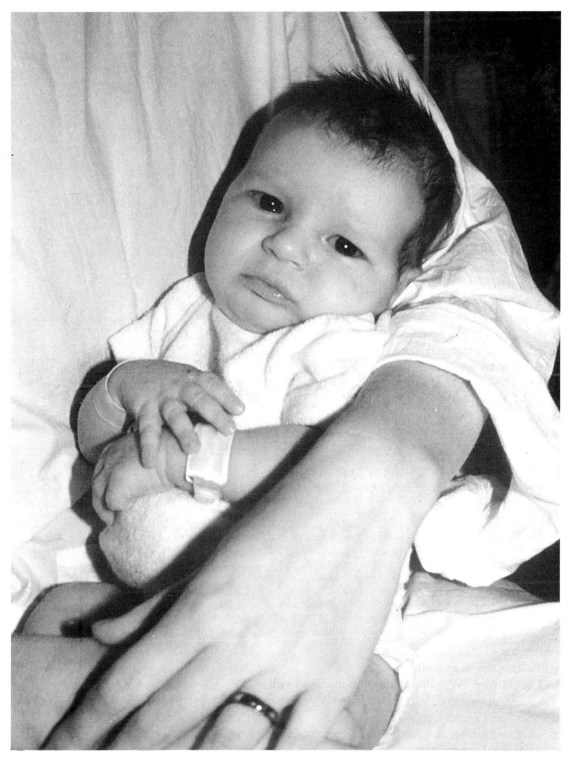

Who should provide the care?

focus in the present study. Yet many aspects of their work will be familiar to nurses generally and especially to those working in other high technology areas.

Actively addressing the problems of staffing and skill-mix from the perspective of the carers can only improve the neonatal unit as a working environment and as a caring environment. Feelings of helplessness on the part of managers and the use of denial as a strategy by senior management reflect the seriousness of the problem. Explanations for the present organisation and structure of neonatal care at regional and trust level are varied. Local conditions, historical precedents and personalities have played their part. Resource allocation has not always been linked effectively with need. Accurate, up-to-date information is required as a basis for this kind of planning and decision-making. The need for a minimum data set has been agreed amongst some of the professionals concerned (BAPM, 1995), but has yet to be in operation in most neonatal units, whose data collection systems vary markedly in quality. The need for rationalization of neonatal services has long been recognised as has the need for a comparable data base that could assist with this (RCP, 1988). While there are units that could be described as "centres of excellence", across the board there is enormous variation and differences persist. Not only is there a lag in responding to recommendations and examples of good practice, there can also be a blindness and lack of vision in relation to change.

The extent to which specific staffing recommendations are in operation could be used as a way of making comparisons between units or between different points in time. The magnitude of differences could be reduced by targeting funding, education and organisational change. Apart from the area of medical staffing, and the introduction of the advanced neonatal nurse practitioner role, the situation in 1994 appears to be little different from that found during the main study period. Large inter-unit differences are still evident that are not related to the needs of babies, parents or staff.

If practice in the area of neonatal care is truly to be "research-based" then the findings of this study like others, must be turned to good effect and utilised. Responses to the research have been varied: regions, health districts, trusts, professional groups and individual nurses and doctors have different perspectives. That other acute services have similar problems and needs (BPA, 1993) in no way diminishes the need to address the issues raised in the area of neonatal care. The study has validated the experience of many neonatal nurses and at the same time resulted in a wealth of information that can be used for measuring change in the specialty and in making comparisons with other areas of nursing.

Conclusion – A Question of Quality

The Strategy for Nursing (DOH, 1989) focused on the major issues of nursing practice, manpower, education, leadership and management.

In A Vision for the Future (DOH, 1993), as in The Patient's Charter (DOH, 1991) and The Health of the Nation (DOH, 1992), nurses, midwives and health visitors are seen as having a key contribution to make towards improvements in health care and the achievement of high quality services. This involves placing the users of the service and their carers at the centre of the service provision, with the aim of providing high quality cost-effective care. The need for partnership and support from managers, doctors and other professional colleagues is emphasised. The vision is one in which care is to be provided on an individual basis, with the outcomes charted and the delivery submitted to audit; clinical and professional leadership will be developed; clinical and professional expertise will feed into the commissioning and purchasing cycle and the educational and personal development needs of practitioners will be met, enabling them to deliver the high quality care required.

How well nursing in the specialty of neonatal care is able to focus on this vision may seem questionable in the context of the study findings. These give rise to a picture of neonatal care that by highlighting the weaknesses and deficiencies may be seen as negative and critical. Yet what also came through in the course of the study was the strength and motivation of nurses working in this specialty. They recognise the value of nursing and their insights, continued dedication and enthusiasm bear witness to their professionalism and hopes for the future. The challenges for neonatal nurses, like nurses in other areas, include innovations in care and organisation, evaluation of change, putting research findings into practice, developing appropriate models of clinical supervision, accountability for practice and clinical and professional leadership. Neonatal nurses are skilled individuals working hard to maintain and improve professional standards. At the time when their babies are in hospital parents are in a dependent role and neonatal nurses act as advocates for them and their babies in many different contexts.

Carers need to be fit for the future and fit for the purpose with appropriate education and support mechanisms in place. In nursing today and particularly in a fast-changing technical specialty like neonatal care a commitment to lifelong learning, institutionally and individually, is required. The rush for degrees shows that many nurses have recognised their own educational needs. Whether or not neonatal or other nurses take on, substitute for or "share" the work of junior doctors, supervision as the cornerstone of clinical practice is the key to setting up and maintaining consistently high standards in relation to care and the clients' needs.

In addition to changing roles, part of the vision for the future is likely to include organisational change and the development of new models of care. As has already happened in a few areas, further links between units, hospitals and trusts will be made as there is rationalisation of the service and some form of accreditation mechanism for intensive care is agreed and established (BAPM, 1995). These moves and changes are all elements in building a seamless web of care of which the neonatal service is part. One possible vision for the future could adopt the model of organisation predicted for neonatal care (Figure 10.1.) in which the roles of the nurses and medical staff participating in the present study have evolved and changed, perhaps beyond the recognition of those currently caring for small sick newborns. The changing boundaries

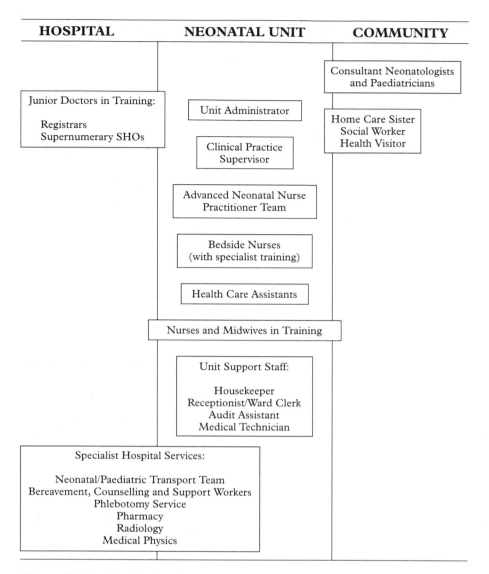

HOSPITAL	NEONATAL UNIT	COMMUNITY

Consultant Neonatologists and Paediatricians

Junior Doctors in Training:

Registrars
Supernumerary SHOs

Unit Administrator

Home Care Sister
Social Worker
Health Visitor

Clinical Practice Supervisor

Advanced Neonatal Nurse Practitioner Team

Bedside Nurses
(with specialist training)

Health Care Assistants

Nurses and Midwives in Training

Unit Support Staff:

Housekeeper
Receptionist/Ward Clerk
Audit Assistant
Medical Technician

Specialist Hospital Services:

Neonatal/Paediatric Transport Team
Bereavement, Counselling and Support Workers
Phlebotomy Service
Pharmacy
Radiology
Medical Physics

Figure 10.1 · Model showing possible future use of medical and nursing staff and other health care workers in neonatal units carrying out intensive care

between the professional groups and between the different types of unit are up for redefinition and to some extent the process has begun (Greenhalge, 1994; Trent Regional Health Authority, 1994; Audit Commission, 1995; Redshaw and Harris, 1995).

The picture of neonatal care created in the course of the research study is a detailed one in which the organisational deficiencies, individual problems and perspectives of parents and staff are integral elements. It is not an area in which every nurse and midwife is willing or able to work. The skills and abilities of those that choose to do so are much needed and valued by parents:

'The best thing was being involved and at the same time knowing my baby was being looked after. If he got into difficulties there was always someone around to help him.'

'We went in one evening. The atmosphere seemed really good, Emma had moved up a room and was out of the incubator – her drips had been removed, she was dressed prettily and wide awake. Both my husband and I felt like crying – it was unbelievable.'

and by neonatal nurses themselves:

'I love my job, especially on a good day. Most of my colleagues are fun, good nurses, supportive and caring. I find work stressful, but perhaps that's why I enjoy neonates.'

References

Audit Commission, (1995) The Doctors' Tale: The work of hospital doctors in England and Wales. HMSO, London.

British Association for Perinatal Medicine, (1995) Standards for Hospitals Providing Neonatal Intensive Care. BAPM, London.

British Paediatric Association, (1993) The Care of Critically Ill Children. Report of Multidisciplinary Working Party on Intensive Care. BPA, London.

DOH, (1989) A Strategy for Nursing: Report of the Steering Committee, HMSO, London.

DOH, (1991) The Patient's Charter, HMSO, London.

DOH, (1992) The Health of the Nation, HMSO, London.

DOH, (1993) A Vision for the Future: The Nursing, Midwifery and Health Visiting Contribution to Health and Health Care. NHSME, HMSO, London.

DOH, (1993/4) Report of the Taskforce on the Strategy for Research in Nursing, Midwifery and Health Visiting. HMSO, London.

Greenhalge and Company, (1994) The Interface Between Junior Doctors and Nurses. Greenhalge, Macclesfield.

Redshaw, M. E. and Harris, A. (1995) An Exploratory Study into the Role of the Advanced Neonatal Nurse Practitioner and the Educational Programme of Preparation. ENB, London.

The Royal College of Physicians, (1988) Medical Care of the Newborn in England and Wales. RCP, London.

Trent Regional Health Authority, (1994) Reduction of Junior Doctors' Hours in Trent Region: The Nursing Contribution. University of Sheffield, 1994.

Delivering Neonatal Care: The Neonatal Unit as a Working Environment: A Survey of Neonatal Nursing

Executive Summary

The Study

An investigation of the organisation and delivery of nursing care in the neonatal service was commissioned by the Department of Health and undertaken by a team from the Department of Child Health in the University of Bristol. The aim was to carry out a major study that could document the present situation and serve as a point of comparison for the future. The findings could also inform policy and identify possible areas for improved management and practice.

Main Points on Organisation and Staffing

- Nurse staffing levels in many units do not match up to the professional standards recommended.

- Large differences exist between units in functional staffing levels.

- Achievement of the recommended levels of staffing is not related to the level of care available or the numbers of designated cots in individual units.

- Some nurses were allocated to care for as many as five babies needing intensive care on one shift. Allocation of two or three intensive care babies and others less dependent was common.

- 58% of nursing staff had worked extra shifts and 43% worked split or long shifts to cover the unit in the previous twelve months.

- Nurse staffing shortages are typically responded to in a short term way, as a reaction to workload fluctuations.

- There is an under-provision of cots in terms of the recommendation of 6 per 1000 live births and an under-funding of intensive care cots in some hospitals.

- 61% of units at times admitted babies requiring intensive care for whom no such designated cots were available.

- The annual staff turnover rate among neonatal nurses was 16% and 8% of posts were vacant at one time. These rates were highest in regional centres.

- In 1990 Medical staffing levels were lower than those recommended in terms of accredited neonatologists, registrars and SHOs.

- By 1994 significant improvements had been made in the medical staffing of neonatal care. Similar improvements were not evident in the area of nurse staffing.

Main Points on Skill Mix

- The largest segment of the neonatal nursing workforce comprises staff nurses and midwives, and of these there are greater numbers of staff nurses.

- Grade E, at 31% was most common, followed by G (19%) and F grades (16%).

- Vacancies were disproportionately high at staff nurse and staff midwife level.

- Skill mix staffing policies were diverse and not clearly related to the type of unit nor the numbers of designated intensive and special care cots.

- More junior grades of staff were employed at night.

- Some unqualified nurses at A and B grades carried out technical and nursing tasks to which qualified staff should be assigned.

- Nursery nurses were employed in 80% of units and all were involved in "hands on" care for babies.

- Nursing auxiliaries were employed in 70% of units and in half of these were involved in "hands on" care of babies.

- The use of support staff, such as ward clerks, technicians and social workers, varied widely and in many units was at very low levels.

Main Points on Education and Training

- 17% of neonatal staff were not registered nurses and only 58% had reached CSE or O-level in their general education.

- The QIS rate at 44%, was less than the 70% aimed at for nurses working in neonatal care. It was highest in the regional centres, followed by sub-regional and district units.

- The QIS rate was highest among sisters and managers, among 30 to 39 year olds and staff rotating between days and nights. It was lowest among the part-time and night staff.

- Neonatal nurses were less mobile than had been expected. Most of the staff (57%) had worked in neonatal care for at least five years or more and 73% had only ever worked in one or two units.

- Orientation programmes for neonatal care are not universal. Only 65% of nurses taking up appointments in the last five years had received them.

- Access to courses and study days was limited. Only 54% of neonatal nursing staff had been on a study day in the last two years.

- More than a quarter of the nursing staff (27%) were waiting to take a post-basic course.

- An appraisal system was said to be in operation by 61% of nurses, but only 47% had been appraised in the last year and 28% not at all.

- 17% of staff had professional development plans.

- Large inter-unit variation was found in QIS rates, even among units of a similar type and size.

Main Points on the Changing Role

- There were large inter-unit differences in the extent to which neonatal nurses have expanded their role.

- Nurses working in neonatal care assist medical staff with a wide range of procedures, including many of those that could be encompassed in an expanded nursing role.

- Some tasks have already been incorporated into the everyday work of qualified nurses in neonatal care. Heel prick blood sampling, removal of IV cannulae and giving IV antibiotics are part of the skill base expected in this area.

- Some experienced senior nurses are now no longer carrying out procedures they have undertaken in the past.

- Senior grade staff and those with a qualification in specialty are more likely to be carrying out "expanded" role tasks.

- A large proportion of nurses graded D-I are routinely undertaking intravenous administration of antibiotics (67%) and of other drugs (50%)

- Relatively few nurses graded D-I are routinely using a blood gas analyser (13%) or a bilirubinometer (12%).

- A small proportion of nurses in neonatal care are regularly carrying out a range of tasks that have more usually been assigned to medical staff, for example removal of chest drain (5%) and IV cannulation (2%).

- A–C grade unit staff caring for babies have carried out some procedures, for example heelprick blood sampling (80%) and removing an IV cannula (52%). More rarely some had undertaken administration of IV antibiotics, removal of an ET tube and removal of an IA cannula.

- Significant numbers of nurses not expanding their practice would like to do so: 51% to give IV drugs other than antibiotics; 63% to site IV cannulae; 71% to intubate; 74% to use a blood gas analyser and 63% to use a bilirubinometer.

- Only small numbers of nurses would like to carry out more invasive procedures such as performing a lumbar puncture (8%) or inserting a chest drain (9%).

Main points on Neonatal Nurses as Working Women

- 83% of the nursing workforce had a partner and 54% had children, with 34% having two or more children.
- 6% of staff took maternity leave in the course of one year and at one point in time 4% were pregnant.
- 75% returned to work in the same neonatal unit after maternity leave: of these 32% returned to their previous duties and the remainder changed from full to part-time work.
- Unit policy varied and in 30% of units nurses changing from full to part-time work were not allowed to keep their grade.
- 5% of managers said job sharing was possible in their unit; 1% of individual nurses were actually working in this way.
- A large proportion of nurses, 43%, worked less than full-time hours. This was more common for those in the lower half of the grading scale and greatest in district units.
- Nursing management varied in the attitude to the employment of part-time nurses: the proportion ranged from 6% to 77% of nurses in a unit.
- 28% of staff worked only at night, most commonly as a function of family commitments.
- Night staff were less likely to be QIS and more likely to be at the lower and cheaper end of the grading scale.
- Workplace nurseries were present in relatively few hospitals and most did not fit in with shift times that neonatal nurses work. Holiday schemes were rare, but considered useful.
- Staff with school age children and children under 5 years of age were likely to have worked longer in neonatal nursing and to have taken less time off sick in the previous three months, than nurses with no children.
- Management attitudes to part-time staff varied and the training needs were felt to be taken less seriously than those of full-time staff in many units.

Main Points on Health and Wellbeing

- The sick leave taken in one year amounted to an average of 9.2. days per nurse employed.
- The reasons given for being ill and taking sick leave included a large proportion of illnesses and conditions thought to be stress-related.
- Neonatal nurses smoke less than the general population and drink as much alcohol.

- Higher sickness rates were associated with larger units and being employed full-time.

- 21% and 10% of neonatal nurses reported themselves as having suffered from anxiety and depression in the last year.

- On a measure of psychological wellbeing 44% of the nursing staff scored above the threshold. With a higher threshold the figure was 33%

- A higher number of life events experienced in the last year were associated with poorer physical and psychological wellbeing.

- The presence of a partner and children appeared to be protective factors.

- Nurses' scores on the measure of psychological wellbeing to some extent correlated with nursing stress levels measured by a standard instrument.

- Neonatal nurses' average stress scores were higher than those reported for a group of urban hospital nurses.

- Stressful incidents and situations were reported by more than 70% of nurses. These covered a small number of topics, predominantly those associated with organisational problems, staffing, sick babies and their parents.

- There were large differences between units in the wellbeing of nursing staff. Support and leadership from senior nursing and medical management was a significant factor in this.

Main Points on Parents' Experience of Neonatal Care Admission

- Babies requiring neonatal care and staying more than two days were commonly those who were preterm or of low birth weight and those with breathing problems.

- Different types of unit have a different case mix: regional centres cared for many of the smallest preterm babies and admitted most of the infants with suspected abnormalities; subregional and district units admitted twice as many babies with hypoglycaemia and a fifth of admissions to district units were associated with feeding problems.

- 20% of babies experienced neonatal care in more than one unit and 6% in three or more hospitals.

Mothers with a baby in a neonatal unit differ from mothers conventionally experiencing a routine delivery and post-natal care:

- 22% of mothers previously had a baby cared for in a neonatal unit.

- 13% of babies were born following an intra-uterine transfer and 17% were transferred subsequently.

- Some babies were born following "at risk" pregnancies, with more than half of the mothers having at least one ante-natal stay in hospital.
- 39% of the study mothers had a caesarean section delivery, most as an emergency, and a further 9% had operative vaginal deliveries.

They may have other concerns too:

- 51% of mothers had other children and 22% had another child of less than two years of age.
- The majority only knew their baby would be admitted to a neonatal unit when they were in labour or at delivery.

Anxiety and distress mark their experience of neonatal care:

- Separation was the worst feature of having a baby admitted to a neonatal unit, and this continued until the baby was discharged home.
- On first seeing their baby in the NNU most parents' main concern was with the baby's appearance and the surrounding equipment. What medical or nursing staff told parents at this time was poorly remembered in comparison.
- Many problems were experienced in visiting a baby in hospital, including the financial costs, the distance and time taken in travelling and having to care for other children at the same time.
- Feeding is one of the most crucial aspects of care in which parents, particularly mothers, can be involved: 55% expressed their own breast milk at least once; 57% of mothers whose babies were tube-fed participated directly at some time and 50% of mothers breastfed or tried to breastfeed in the neonatal unit.
- Insufficient advice, information, support and privacy were key issues for breast and bottle feeding mothers.

Variation between units was evident:

- Large inter-unit differences were found in the extent to which the development of parenting skills were actively encouraged and facilitated.
- Visiting policies differed without a clear rationale and were not apparently related to parental need.
- Antenatal visits to the neonatal unit as part of the preparation for parenthood is not routine. 58% of units had such a policy in operation, but only 20% of mothers had seen the unit before their baby was born.
- Parents were allowed to stay for ward rounds in 75% of units, but in the remainder they were asked to leave.

- The information available varied enormously: less than half the units had their own information booklet and 40% had no booklet at all; only half had a board with photographs and names identifying staff.
- Facilities also varied widely: conditions were extremely cramped in some units; very few had a playroom for siblings to use; most had a sitting room and overnight accommodation for parents, but the quality of these varied greatly and rooms were sometimes shared with nursing and medical staff.

For parents whose baby was terminally ill or whose baby had died the situation appeared to be improving:

- There was generally great sensitivity and awareness of the needs of parents in this situation in many units specific guidelines were being developed and followed.
- A quiet room to be with the baby, a crib or moses basket, photographs and keepsakes were available and used by almost all the bereaved parents.
- Comments from bereaved parents about their experience emphasised the need for better communication, greater honesty, and the need to be listened to and not hurried.

Recommendations

Organisation and Staffing

- Positive steps to ensure staffing levels are improved to meet more recent recommended levels.
- A more flexible mechanism for updating the establishment and calculating staffing needs. A formula that fully takes account of workload, vacancies, sick and maternity leave, educational and compassionate leave requirements.
- Regular, at least annual, reviews of nursing establishment in relation to workload are needed that are based on adequate data collection and collation.
- More experienced SHOs and better neonatal training and supervision for them, or other appropriately qualified staff to take on their duties. Middle-grade medical staff are needed in those few units without them.
- Neonatologists in all regional and subregional centres.
- Accreditation of units for intensive and high dependency care.

Nursing Skill Mix

- A re-examination of the skill requirements in the context of neonatal care.

- The same core mixture of skilled and experienced staff to be employed in caring for babies on all three shifts.

- A reassessment of the role of junior nursing staff, especially in relation to intensive care and high dependency babies,

- Wider employment of support staff: medical technicians and unit-based social workers in all regional and sub-regional centres, and adequate numbers of ward clerks in all types of unit on day and evening shifts.

Training and Education

- A more positive attitude and proactive management strategy directed towards staff training and update for all levels of nursing staff is needed.

- More opportunities for staff to become qualified in the specialty of neonatal nursing are required. Funding for courses should be related to need, so that the present inter-unit differences in levels of QIS do not persist.

- More courses geared to increasing the numbers of part-time and night staff with a qualification in specialty.

- Increased awareness and response to the need for management training for the senior neonatal unit staff.

- A more professional approach on the part of individual members of staff and management is required in the area of staff appraisal and career development.

Neonatal Nurses as Working Women

- The needs of neonatal nurses as working women demand to be addressed directly and coherently in a number of ways Maternity leave requirements must adequately be taken into account in calculating staffing needs, the implication of changing shift patterns considered and the question of more workable forms of child care investigated.

- Many part-time staff and nurses with children are currently caring for babies in neonatal units. Training and update programmes that include them and facilitate their participation should be encouraged and developed.

- Retention strategies should include more flexible working arrangements that allow temporary adjustments in response to changing personal circumstances.

Health and Sickness

- Greater awareness of how an individuals' health can be affected by stress is needed. Teaching on this should be an integral element in training courses for neonatal nurses

- The development of appropriate counselling and support services, including those concerned with bereavement.

- Recognition of the contributory problem of staff shortages and high workload demands.

- An attempt should be made by the profession as a whole to address the problems encountered by older staff in a fast-changing, technical specialty.

Parents and Families

- More antenatal preparation regarding neonatal care.

- Increased awareness of the needs and problems of mothers following caesarean section or operative delivery.

- More information, presented in a variety of forms is needed for parents with a baby in neonatal care.

- Involvement of both parents in caring for their baby needs to be actively encouraged, even from an early stage.

- A more widespread positive attitude towards breastfeeding.

- Privacy should be available and offered to parents, especially for breastfeeding.

- Parents need to be made aware of the facilities available.

- Neonatal units should have a sitting room for parents and overnight accommodation that is not shared with medical staff.

- In some units visiting policies require rationalisation so that parents can have a choice about who accompanies them to visit.

- Better communication is needed between units, especially those involved in transferring babies.

- The role of the "family care sister" should be developed in the context of closer links between hospitals and the community.

- Training and support is needed for staff dealing with bereaved parents.

Conclusion

While the last two decades have seen the situation in neonatal care improve for sick babies and their families, less has changed in the area of organisation and staffing. Much innovation will be needed if the issues raised directly and indirectly in the course of this study are to be addressed.

Abbreviations

ANNP	Advanced Neonatal Nurse Practitioner
BPA	British Paediatric Association
BAPM	British Association of Perinatal Medicine
BP	Blood Pressure
C405	ENB Course 405
CNM	Clinical Nurse Manager
CNS	Clinical Nurse Specialist
CNT	Clinical Nurse Teacher
CSAG	Clinical Standards Advisory Group
CVP	Central Venous Pressure
DHSS	Department of Health and Social Security
DOH	Department of Health
EN	Enrolled Nurse
ENB	English National Board for Nursing, Midwifery and Health Visiting
ETT	Endotracheal Tube
gm	Gramme
IA	Intra-arterial
IM	Intramuscular
IV	Intravenous
IPPV	Intermittent Positive Pressure Ventilation
JBCNS	Joint Board of Clinical Nursing Studies
LP	Lumbar Puncture
NAux	Nursing Auxiliary
NHSME	National Health Service Management Executive
NICU	Neonatal Intensive Care Unit
NNA	Neonatal Nurses Association
NN	Nursery Nurse
NNU	Neonatal Unit
O$_2$	Oxygen
QIS	Qualification in Specialty
RCP	Royal College of Physicians
RN	Registered Nurse
RM	Registered Midwife
RSCN	Registered Sick Childrens Nurse
SCBU	Special Care Baby Unit

SM	Staff Midwife
SN	Staff Nurse
SR	Sister
UAC	Umbilical Arterial Catheter
UKCC	United Kingdom Central Council for Nursing, Midwifery and Health Visiting
WTE	Whole Time Equivalent

Glossary of Terms Used

Arterial blood pressure monitoring
Continual monitoring of mean, systolic and diastolic blood pressure via an indwelling cannula or catheter using a pressure sensitive monitoring device.

Bag and mask
Device used for delivering air and/or oxygen under pressure via the patients nose and mouth to the airways.

Bank nurse
A nurse temporarily supplied to a unit who is willing to work hours on nominated days.

Bilirubinometer
Laboratory equipment used to estimate serum bilirubin levels.

Blood gas analyser
Laboratory equipment for analysing pH, oxygen, carbon dioxide and bicarbonate content of blood samples.

Blood sampling
Intermittent collection of blood specimens obtained from heelprick, venepuncture, arterial stab or withdrawal from indwelling arterial or venous line.

Bronchial lavage
Introduction of saline into the main bronchus under direct vision using a laryngoscope, with the aim of loosening secretions which are removed by mechanical suction.

Case-mix
Mixture of patients with different presenting or subsequent problems.

Central or long line
Passage of a fine silastic catheter using a scalp vein, medial antecubital, long saphenous or subclavian vein. The aim is to position the catheter just inside the right atrium to give long-term intravenous fluids or feeds.

Chest drain
Fine plastic thoracentesis tube inserted via the second and third intercostal space. When secured in position and connected to a hemlich valve or underwater seal system allows the drainage of a pneumothorax to take place.

Clinical Grading
Career progression ladder for nurses (A–I) linked to responsibilities and qualification introduced in 1988.

Clinical procedures
Practical, often invasive techniques carried out in connection with life-saving, diagnostic or treatment measures.

Competence
Stage of development characterised by an increased level of efficiency.

Competency
A defined area of skilled performance identified and described by its purpose, functions and meanings.

Controlled drugs
Medications covered by the Misuse of Drugs Act 1971.

Endotracheal tube
Plastic tube graduated in length and available in various sizes for placing in the trachea to provide respiratory support.

English National Board for Nursing, Midwifery and Health Visiting
Statutory body charged with validation and control of pre and post-registration nurse education.

Extubation
Removal of endotracheal tube from the bronchus.

Health Care Assistant
Support staff recruited to replace the traditional nurse learner contribution.

High-technology
Large amount of technical equipment.

Indwelling cannula
Fine PVC or teflon coated tube inserted into a peripheral vein (intravenous) or an artery (intr-arterial) and secured in situ to provide venous/arterial access.

Intermittent positive pressure ventilation
Mechanical ventilation of the lungs providing air and/or additional oxygen under positive pressure and within pre-set parameters.

Intubation
Passage of endotracheal tube via the naso or oropharynx through the larynx and into the trachea to ventilate the lungs.

Junior doctors
House officers, Senior House Officers, Registrars and Senior Registrars.

Lumbar puncture
Introduction of a disposable needle between the 3rd and 4th lumbar vertebrae to the subarachnoid space. Cerebrospinal fluid is collected for diagnostic purposes.

Named Nurse
A specific nurse allocated to oversee the care of a particular baby and family throughout a hospital stay.

Neonatal
The first 28 days of life.

Neonatal Intensive Care
Continuous skilled supervision of newborn babies (up to 28 days old and longer if necessary) by qualified and specifically trained nursing and medical staff involving assisted ventilation and/or specialised procedures other than ventilation.

Neonatal units
Hospital departments which provide intensive and/or special care for babies.

Nursing establishment
Number of staff at each grade funded in the unit staffing budget. Measured in whole-time equivalents.

Nursing Process
A systematic problem solving approach to patient care.

Peritoneal dialysis
Cyclic administration and drainage of specific dialysis fluid into the peritoneum via a catheter as treatment for renal failure and other problems.

Philosophy of care
A statement drawn up by unit staff of the aims of patient care specific to the types of babies usually cared for in their unit.

Phlebotomy service
Laboratory support staff responsible for the routine collection of blood samples from patients.

Policy
Written document containing agreed methods of action in particular situations.

Primary Nursing
Nursing philosophy and organisation of care where a 'primary nurse' is nominated to care for each baby and family on admission, then assumes 24-hour responsibility and authority for all aspects of nursing care throughout the hospital stay.

Protocol
Statement giving detailed direction on how to carry out specific activities or procedures in accordance with the requirements of a particular institution.

Post-registration
Considered as the period following initial nurse training.

Qualification in specialty
Possession of ENB Course 405, 904 or earlier versions of these.

Sampling intra-arterial
Intermittent collection of arterial blood sample via an indwelling cannula or lines catheter.

Skill mix
Mixture of different levels of nursing staff employed in a particular clinical area.

Supra-pubic
Introduction of needle into the bladder via the pubic region to obtain an **aspiration** uncontaminated sample of urine for diagnostic purposes.

Task allocation
Organisation of nursing work using tasks to undertake rather than whole patients to care for.

Team nursing
Allocation of nurses to care for groups of babies and families for a number of shifts.

Total parenteral nutrition
Solutions given intravenously to replace or supplement enteral feeding requirements. Containing mixtures of proteins, fat emulsions, carbohydrates, vitamins and minerals.

Tube feeding
Milk feed given via a syringe and fine tube which is passed into the stomach or jejunum via the oro or naso-pharynx. The feed may be given as a bolus intermittently or continuously by a pump.

Umbilical arterial catheter
PVC catheter passed via the umbilical artery. Once sutured in situ the catheter is used for blood sampling, fluid administration or blood pressure monitoring.

United Kingdom Central Council for Nursing Midwifery and Health Visiting
The professional body charged with control of registration and standards in nursing, midwifery and health visiting.

Ventilator
Mechanical equipment used to maintain flow of air and/or oxygen into and out of the lungs within set parameters.

Ventricular tap
Passage of fine needle under ultrasound control through the anterior fontanelle into the ventricle. Usually to relieve intercranial pressure due to an accumulation of cerebrospinal fluid.

Very low birthweight babies
Less than 1500 grammes at birth.

Index

Entries refer to neonatal nursing/nurses unless otherwise specified. Page numbers in bold denote executive summary. f denotes figure. t denotes table.

Printed in the United Kingdom for HMSO
Dd301270 5/96 C15 G559 10170